GP WELLBEING

Combatting Burnout in General Practice

GP WELLBEING

Combatting Burnout in
General Practice

Adam Staten
Euan Lawson

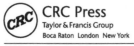

CRC Press
Taylor & Francis Group
Boca Raton London New York

CRC Press is an imprint of the
Taylor & Francis Group, an **informa** business

CRC Press
Taylor & Francis Group
6000 Broken Sound Parkway NW, Suite 300
Boca Raton, FL 33487-2742

© 2018 by Taylor & Francis Group, LLC
CRC Press is an imprint of Taylor & Francis Group, an Informa business

No claim to original U.S. Government works

Printed in Great Britain by Ashford Colour Press Ltd

International Standard Book Number-13: 978-1-1380-6634-2 (Hardback)
978-1-1380-6627-4 (Paperback)

Library of Congress Cataloging-in-Publication Data

Names: Staten, Adam, author. | Lawson, Euan, author.
Title: GP wellbeing : combatting burnout in general practice / Adam Staten, Euan Lawson.
Description: Boca Raton : CRC Press, [2018] | Includes bibliographical references and index.
Identifiers: LCCN 2017034018 (print) | LCCN 2017034987 (ebook) | ISBN 9781315159218 (Master eBook) | ISBN 9781138066342 (hardback : alk. paper) | ISBN 9781138066274 (paperback : alk. paper)
Subjects: | MESH: General Practitioners | Burnout, Professional--prevention & control | Adaptation, Psychological | Job Satisfaction | General Practice | United Kingdom
Classification: LCC R118 (ebook) | LCC R118 (print) | NLM WB 110 | DDC 610--dc23
LC record available at https://lccn.loc.gov/2017034018

Visit the Taylor & Francis Web site at
http://www.taylorandfrancis.com

and the CRC Press Web site at
http://www.crcpress.com

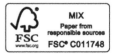

Contents

Preface

INTRODUCTION

The phenomenon of doctors becoming overwhelmed by the stresses of their job is not new, but in recent years burnout has become an enormous issue in UK general practice. The many accumulated stresses of life as a general practitioner (GP) are taking their toll and are causing nothing short of a workforce crisis.

A survey of more than 2000 National Health Service (NHS) GPs conducted by the journal *Pulse* in 2015 found that 50% of them thought that they were at high risk of burnout. This figure had risen from 46% just 2 years previously. A Commonwealth Fund survey conducted in the same year found that 29% of UK GPs wanted to leave the profession within 5 years, and yet more were unsure whether their long-term future lay in general practice. At a time when the NHS needs more GPs than ever, it is instead haemorrhaging doctors at an ever-increasing rate.

The workload of general practice seems to be increasing inexorably, reportedly increasing by 16% in the past 7 years. In 2013, GPs provided more than 340 million patient consultations, a rise of 40 million from 2008, and this accounted for 90% of patient contacts within the NHS. The Conservative government elected in 2015 made a commitment to provide 5000 more GPs by 2020 to help relieve the pressure, but with falling recruitment, early retirement and many doctors simply walking away from clinical practice in the middle of their careers, this looks like an unachievable aim.

Worryingly, half of GP leavers are younger than 50 years old and 77% of those planning on switching career are younger than 55 years old. It seems that GPs are burning out quickly and burning out young.

CAN IT REALLY BE THAT BAD?

General practice remains the last bastion of medical generalism in a world of increasing specialisation. Unlike our secondary care colleagues who work in ever-narrowing fields, general practice is a cornucopia of physical and mental pathology, and one of the few places in medicine where doctors come at symptomatology and disease fresh while it is untainted by the investigations and treatments of others. It is only in general practice that care can be truly holistic and where we have the privilege of caring continuously for our patients over decades. It is a place where we can make a real difference to our patients' lives, not just to their illnesses.

More than this, there is enormous and exciting variety within general practice. No two GPs need work in the same way because GPs are in universal demand in environments as diverse as isolated Scottish Islands, to inner city addiction clinics, from battlefields where they administer care to battlefield trauma, to research institutions where they conduct cutting-edge research. With extended roles, special interests, opportunities to be entrepreneurial or political, a career in general practice can be what you want it to be. Broadly trained and adaptable, GPs are also well placed to respond to the ever changing world of the NHS.

But something seems to be stopping GPs thriving in this world of possibilities. Why can 29% of our colleagues not imagine themselves continuing to work in general practice for another 5 years? How is it that 25% of GPs feel that the stress of their job has made them unwell within the past 12 months?

This book is an attempt to understand why we are in this situation, what factors have brought us here and how we can change the system, our careers and, perhaps, ourselves to cope with the stresses of our jobs.

This book explores the problems of NHS general practice, some of which are systemic and some of which are individual. We discuss the administrative and political burdens of general practice and the issues caused by the rising demands placed on GPs by an enlarging, ageing and increasingly poly-morbid population. We explore the possible solutions to these problems, some of which require the system to change, and some that are based on changes that individuals can make for themselves.

In response to the pressures that they face, GPs around the country are already working innovatively and collaboratively to overcome them, and this book discusses new proposals to change the way we consult, the way we structure our primary health care teams, the way in which we use technology and the way we interact with our secondary care colleagues.

Working GPs explain how diversifying their careers and finding niches for themselves working within academia, or with refugees, or in remote locations, has helped to keep their careers satisfying and fulfilling. And the nature of burnout, the nature of resilience and what can be done to prevent burnout and encourage resilience are discussed.

What we hope is demonstrated by the end of the final chapter is that in this crisis there is a great deal of opportunity. There is the opportunity to improve our working lives and to improve the way we deliver care to our patients.

Working independently and on a relatively small scale, the UK GP is uniquely placed within the NHS to act dynamically and change things rapidly to suit both doctors and patients. An increasing level of GP burnout is not inevitable, but it is probable unless we seek out its root causes and act now to counter them.

Adam Staten
The Red House Surgery, Bletchley

Euan Lawson
Lancaster University

Introduction

The term 'burnout' was created in 1974 by the psychologist Herbert Freudenberger who described job dissatisfaction precipitated by work-related stress.[1] The most common measure of burnout is the Maslach Burnout Inventory (MBI) used for the past 25 years.[2] This defines and measures burnout in three domains: *emotional exhaustion* (feelings of being emotionally overextended and exhausted by one's work), *depersonalisation* (an unfeeling and impersonal response to those who receive the individual's services, treatment or instruction) and *personal accomplishment* (feelings of incompetence in one's work). The World Health Organization's International Classification defines burnout as a 'state of vital exhaustion'.[3]

However, one defines burnout, it is recognised as a state of *emotional, mental and physical exhaustion caused by long-term involvement in emotionally demanding situations* and where the individual cannot, for whatever reason, meet the constant demands placed upon them.[4] Burnout is therefore best thought of as a spectrum of symptoms ranging from tearfulness, depersonalisation, feelings of hopelessness, depression and anxiety (in some cases indistinguishable from depression). It might in fact be a more acceptable, less stigmatizing label for health professionals to accept than depression.

Burnout is ubiquitous. In all health systems, age or length of practice, approximately 50% of doctors meet the criteria for burnout at any one time. In some populations, for example, younger doctors' rates can reach as high as 70%. Surveys over the past 20 years have consistently shown that, on average, around one-third of doctors are suffering from burnout at any one time, worldwide, regardless of specialty. In a 2012 survey by the Physician's Foundation, 60% of US physicians reported they would retire immediately if they could. The 2014 Medscape Physician's Lifestyle Survey showed a 46% prevalence of at least one symptom of burnout in a responder group of 20,000 American physicians.[5]

Given the nature of medicine, its emotional demands and the need to put patients first, it could be said that burnout is an occupational hazard of being a doctor. However, burnout seems to be getting worse. For example, the 7th National General Practitioner (GP) Work Life Survey found the lowest levels of job satisfaction and the highest levels of stress since the beginning of the National GP Worklife Survey. It also found the highest level of GPs expecting to quit – especially in those over 50 years old (54.1%).[6]

PRACTITIONER HEALTH

For about a decade I have been the medical director of the Practitioner Health Programme (www.php.nhs.uk), a confidential service for doctors in London with mental health and addiction problems. Since January 2017, the service has been extended to all GPs in England (called GP Health Service, www. gphealth.nhs.uk). Over the decade, the service has seen more than 3000 doctors presenting (this around 10% of all doctors in London). Most have common mental health problems – depression, anxiety and symptoms indistinguishable from post-traumatic stress disorder. All specialties have presented. GPs, paediatricians and emergency care doctors are over-represented. Surgeons are under-represented – more likely a hidden minority group within a hidden minority. Around one-third of the doctors have problems with addiction, mostly alcohol.

Over the years, the age of the doctors presenting to the service has dropped from a median age of 50 years (2009) to a median age of 29 years (2011). Of course, not all mental health problems in doctors are related to their work; for example, doctors are exposed to the same external life events as non-doctors and are not immune to marital breakup, illness, loss and other common life events. However, work plays an important part in a doctor's life and for many defines who they are. Given this, it is hardly surprising that doctors who attend specialist sick-doctor services do so late in their illness, often in a crisis or after a problem at work or drink-drive offence. They literally work to the bitter end. Even when the signs of mental illness are obvious, doctors find it difficult to leave work behind them and even harder to seek the help they so readily prescribe for their patients. Doctors also have barriers in seeking help. These include practical difficulties, for example, taking time out to make an appointment, or where they might live and work in the same area and have to see someone they know professionally or personally. There are financial implications for self-employed doctors taking time off sick, as even if insured most policies do not commence until at least 1-month sickness absence and are unlikely to cover the full costs of locum cover.

Stigma in accepting a mental health diagnosis is particularly common amongst doctors, and high levels of self-stigmatisation represent a major obstacle to accessing healthcare and, once unwell, returning to work. The 'stiff upper lip' is alive and well in the profession. When doctors do approach services, staff and patients can treat them differently, adding to the isolation already felt by a mentally ill doctor. GPs might deny their vulnerability and not want to be seen as the weak link in their teams – especially where they might be leading teams. Fears that they might be referred to the General Medical Council if they admit to having more serious mental health issues such as bipolar disorder or alcohol or drug dependence also act as obvious barriers to seeking help.

WORK AND MEANING AS A RISK FACTOR FOR BURNOUT

Both mental illness and burnout are more common in those working in the caring professions, especially where high degrees of altruism, self-sacrifice and making others (namely patients) the main concern are required. Doctors are at risk because their job defines them and gives a sense of meaning to life. Even before arriving at medical school the embryonic doctor is embedded into a profession which (implicitly or explicitly) sees itself as 'special'. From medical school onward, students learn, play, work, live and even love together, creating a deep-rooted 'medical self' or 'vocation', which incorporates the personal and the professional selves into a single persona. The person becomes the doctor, the doctor becomes the person. Inseparable. Goffman-esque as a total profession, doctors spend most waking hours in the bounded space of their medical space, which defines and contains them through their work; unable to leave behind at the end of the day, as one doctor said, *the hospital almost replaces your family.....being a medic is not just a job that you go to, but something you are.*

During training, doctors learn a unique scientific language and symbolically the medical-self, contained within the medical world, is re-enforced through dress (the white coat, albeit worn less and less), and especially through the acquisition of a new name: 'doctor', institutionalising their sense of being special.[7] Every success and failure is personalised; as long as the involvement, commitment and hard work are rewarded by continuous success (no matter how small), doctors gain a sense of meaning from their work, and this becomes a virtuous circle.

CAUSES OF BURNOUT

Burnout occurs when it is impossible to achieve anymore; when inadequate resources or lack of autonomy makes it impossible to accomplish work goals and frustration erodes the spirit. Given the nature of medicine, doctors are always going to fail (as they cannot cure all illness, alleviate all pain or stop death) and hence burnout is inevitable.

Summary of causes of burnout	
Work related	Having little or no control over work
	Lack of recognition or reward for good work
	Unclear or overly demanding job expectations
	Doing work that is monotonous or unchallenging
	Working in a chaotic or high-pressure environment
Lifestyle	Poor sleep
	Working too much, without enough time for socialising or relaxing
	Lack of close, supportive relationships
	Taking on too many responsibilities, without enough help from others

Continued

Summary of causes of burnout	
Personality traits	Perfectionistic tendencies; nothing is ever good enough
	Pessimism
	Need to be in control; reluctance to delegate to others
	High-achieving, competitive personality
Socio-political	Societies' unrealistic expectations of what doctors can do with medicine, leading to doctors being the container for fear, anxiety and disappointment
	Funding pressures, unable to achieve the care promised by governmental bodies

Burnout is not entirely due to pressures of the job or training. Doctors are more at risk because *they are chosen* for those personality factors which foster the antecedents of burnout, and these factors also attract them to a career in medicine, for example, altruism, perfectionism and obsessiveness. A compulsive triad of doubt, guilt and exaggerated sense of responsibility, again common amongst doctors, adds to this vulnerability.[8] Over the course of training and later work, doctors develop defences to counter these characteristics.

In the 1950s the sociologist Menzies-Lyth described how it is necessary to develop defences, such as depersonalisation and denial of feelings to work in proximity to death, despair and disease.[9] Her observations of student nurses showed that the anxiety caused by close and intimate involvement with patients' illnesses and deaths could be avoided through the development of social defences – social as they were created by the organisation, vicariously protecting the individuals within the system. Defences such as discouraging attachment and engagement with a patient by constantly moving nurses from ward to ward or breaking down patient care into smaller and smaller 'production line' tasks undertaken by different individuals and finally defences such as encouraging depersonalisation by referring to the patient in abstract ways such as 'the liver in bed 10'.

Of course, health professionals must be able to detach themselves from their patients, not to over-identify with them and to be able to drop their mask of empathy at times. But the defences which protect from becoming over engaged with patients also, and especially where there is no time to reflect on our failures or meet with peers, can turn against the carer.

EFFECTS OF BURNOUT

For some doctors this results in disengagement and increasing aggression against 'the other', be this the patient, the employer or the NHS. They present with problems at work, a complaint from a patient or member of staff. Or doctors become increasingly detached from their teams and become psychological isolates, unable to give to anyone other than their patients. These doctors ignore the needs of their families and friends or even ignore important professional or personal deadlines. These doctors may fail to pay bills or meet the requirements for appraisal or revalidation, or they may experience boundary violations with patients.

For other doctors, they deal with their anxiety by working harder, staying longer and longer at work and taking on an excessive sense of responsibility for things beyond their control; 'it must be my fault' combined with the chronic feelings of 'not doing enough'. These doctors present with anxiety or depression and guilt for not caring enough and shame for not being able to meet the needs of their patients. Unaddressed, and with added vulnerabilities, burnout for all doctors can lead to substance misuse, depression, anxiety and suicide.

BURNOUT IN CONTEXT

Burnout is not new. A classic book in the history of general practice is John Berger's *A Fortunate Man: The Story of a Country Doctor*.[10] This book describes the real-life story of the heroic and caring GP, John Sassall. What is clear from John Sassall is that he was far from a role model we should aspire to. Like many of the doctors in modern practice, he gave his all to his patients, combined his personal and professional selves and blurred the boundaries between his professional and private lives. Far from being a celebration of a time lost, of an era of general practice that we should aspire to, it should become compulsory reading on how to prevent the balance tilting toward burnout. Sassall, too, was a single-handed GP in the Forest of Dean. He had been a dual-handed practitioner for many years, but when his long-term partner died, instead of acquiring a new partner, he instead split the list and became single handed. Sassall was a workaholic. He relished his work. It gave him meaning. The book describes how he longed to be woken at night to do house calls. That he was incapable of doing nothing, and just being. Sassall becomes deeply depressed, so much so that his reactions were slowed and his concentration reduced – but so dedicated or more likely lacking in insight, work he did. Sassall ended his own life.

The psychotherapist Carl Jung described the paradigm of the wounded healer and the archetype of *those who care for others, out of vocation or compulsion, often masking the difficulties in caring for themselves.* This characteristic is hinted at in *A Fortunate Man*, when Berger wrote that Sassall *cures others to cure himself…* in essence denying his own vulnerability by creating dependence in his patients and vicariously healing himself through them. Burnout, or as with Sassal, depression, is therefore not new, and neither will it ever go away – it is an inevitable consequence of working so close to patients. We are better served by thinking of burnout as being at one end of a balance and mental wellbeing at the other; we should aim over our professional life to shift the balance toward the latter through personal and organisational interventions. And between supporting the individual and bringing about changes in the prevailing culture.

TOWARD A UNIFYING SOLUTION

There is a sense that the increase in burnout is due to the current generation of doctors being less resilient than those of previous generations. However, it is my view that all generations of doctors are remarkably resilient. Doctors, past and present, are amongst the most resilient individuals in society – they can go long hours without sleep, food and bathroom breaks (they even have resilient bladders). Doctors survive and thrive and adapt in the face of adversity. Resilience is about bending with pressure and bouncing back. But given the right (or wrong) environmental factors, a storm, fire or undue pressure, everyone will have their elastic limit and will break – some will develop burnout and the more vulnerable will develop depression, anxiety, substance misuse or other mental health problems. More regulation, less time to care, marketised and industrialised health systems and increasing litigation all add to the environmental or prevailing pressures.

DEALING WITH BURNOUT

Most doctor-directed interventions involve mindfulness, behavioural treatment, mentoring, coaching or addressing personal coping strategies.[11] On the whole, direct time and attention to any doctor and this will help – and the evidence shows this, irrespective of the modality the outcome is the same – improvement with attention.[12,13]

Going forward, we must not fall into the trap of locating the disturbance just in the individual or individual practice as this separates the individual from the wider environmental stresses. Instead, we need a three-pronged approach.

The first approach is related to the *individual*: What can 'I' do: How can I create a balance in my life between play and work? What can I do to reduce my individual stressors or recharge my psychological batteries? Research shows that simple interventions, such as taking holidays; having time with friends or family; sport, music or simply just standing still, help reduce burnout. For each of us as well, it is important to realise our limits and when things seem to be going wrong, or when our mood dips or we feel that we are resorting to unhealthy coping strategies, then think about seeking help.

The second approach is what can *teams* do: What can 'we' do? This is about addressing our workplace and examining ways of reducing stressors where we can, such as looking at rotas, adding in breaks between patients and looking at the spaces where we can meet to learn or reflect together. Medicine is a relational activity – and increasingly the spaces where doctors (and other health professionals) meet together for formal and informal meetings are rapidly disappearing. Putting in spaces for groups, either daily 15-min micro-meetings or weekly 60-min team meetings or monthly 90-min reflective practice groups, has been shown to reduce the risk of burnout. Organisational factors, including addressing work pressure, resources (time, people and money) and spaces and opportunities for team working, are probably more important and evidence shows more likely to make a difference.

Finally, going forward it is important to address the macro-*environmental* and external causes of distress: What can 'they' do? The 'they' being those who build the regulatory, financial, organisational and investigation systems in which we work. Addressing these massive structures involves policy makers, politicians and senior leaders understanding that without structural change even the most resilient individual will break. It means addressing factors, such as regulatory requirements, political influences and media pressures.

Balance work and play (between the machinery of caring and actual
caring, declutter the space in the consulting room between us and
our patients)
Understand our limitations – we are not superheroes
Recognise, prevent and treat burnout in ourselves and our teams
Nurture the next generation – bring the fun back into work
Teamwork (working in groups, restore the times and spaces to work,
rest, play and reflect together)

Finally, burnout is common and a normal aspect of a doctor's work. Going forward, doctors have to learn to identify it and manage it throughout their professional lives.

Dr. Clare Gerada
Medical Director Practitioner Health: Principle General Practice
Former Chair of the Royal College of General Practitioners

REFERENCES

1. Freudenberger HJ. Staff burnout. *J Soc Issues* 1974;30(1):159–65.
2. Maslach C. Burnout: A multidimensional perspective. In Schaufeli WB, Maslach C, Marek T, editors. *Professional burnout: Recent developments in theory and research.* Washington, DC: Taylor & Francis; 1993.
3. World Health Organization. *International Statistical Classification of Diseases and Related Health Problems.* 10th Rev. (ICD-10). Geneva: World Health Organization; 2004.
4. Beck R, Buchele B. In the belly of the beast: Traumatic countertransference. *Int J Group Psychother* 2005;55(1):31–44.
5. *The Physicians Foundation a Survey of America's Physicians.* 2012. http://www.physiciansfoundation.org/uploads/default/Physicians_ Foundation_2012_Biennial_Survey.pdf. Accessed on 19 July, 2017.
6. Hann M, McDonald J, Checkland K, Coleman A, Gravelle H, Sibbald B, Sutton M. *Seventh National GP Worklife Survey.* http://www.population-health.manchester.ac.uk/healtheconomics/research/reports/FinalReportof the7thNationalGPWorklifeSurvey.pdf. Accessed on 19 July, 2017.
7. Wessely A, Gerada C. *When doctors need treatment: An anthropological approach to why doctor make bad patients.* http://careers.bmj.com/ careers/advice/view-article.html?id=20015402. Accessed on 19 July, 2017.
8. Gabbard O. The role of compulsiveness in the normal physician. *JAMA* 1985;254(20):2926–9. doi: 10.1001/jama.1985.03360200078031.
9. Menzies Lyth I. The functions of social systems as a defence against anxiety: A report on a study of the nursing service of a general hospital. *Hum Relat* 1959;13:95–121; reprinted *in Containing Anxiety in Institutions: Selected Essays, vol. 1.* Free Association Books, 1988, pp. 43–88.

10. Berger J. *A fortunate man: The story of a country doctor.* London: RCGP; 2005.
11. West C, Durbye L, Erwin P, Shanafelt T. Interventions to prevent and reduce physician burnout: A systematic review and meta-analysis. *Lancet* 2016;388:2272–81.
12. Panagioti M, Panagopoulou E, Bower P, Lewith G, Kontopantelis E, Chew-Graham C, Dawson S, van Marwijk H, Geraghty K, Esmail A. Controlled interventions to reduce burnout in physicians. A systematic review and meta-analysis. *JAMA Intern Med* 2017;177(2):195–205. doi: 10.1001/jamainternmed.2016.7674.
13. Nielsen H, Tulinius C. Preventing burnout among general practitioners: Is there a possible route? *Educ Primary Care* 2009;20:353–9.

1

What is burnout?

DR. ADAM STATEN
The Red House Surgery, Bletchley, UK

Burnout is more than feeling stressed. Burnout is a pervasive and debilitating state that results from an unsustainable period of overwhelming stress. It is not a new phenomenon. The term was coined by the psychologist Herbert Freudenberger in 1974 who recognised the condition in himself and colleagues whilst working in drug addiction clinics in New York.[1] Nor is burnout limited to those working in health care.[2] It is a familiar concept in many areas of life from the financial services sector to professional sports.

Increasingly, burnout is recognised as a widespread issue in modern life, and this pervasiveness is reflected by the deluge of new research that is being conducted on burnout, not to mention the abundance of self-help literature that is published every year to assist people in coping with stress and burnout, whatever the cause. Burnout seems to be especially common amongst those in caring professions such as health care, social work and teaching, with a prevalence of up to 25% in these professions suggested by some research.[3]

In particular, burnout amongst general practitioners (GPs) working within the National Health Service (NHS) seems to be on the rise, and this is causing problems not just for the individuals concerned, but for a health care system that is reliant on having a healthy, happy and functional primary care workforce. Thus, it is essential that we as individuals, and the system as a whole, understand what burnout is, what impact it has and how it can be stopped.

KEY FEATURES OF BURNOUT

Burnout is classically defined as an experience of physical, emotional and mental exhaustion caused by long-term involvement with situations that are emotionally demanding.[3] It comprises three major components: emotional exhaustion, depersonalisation and an absent sense of personal accomplishment.[4] These three major components were incorporated into a scoring system, the Maslach Burnout

1

Inventory, which has been used to evaluate and study burnout in a variety of settings, and in a variety of guises, since its creation in 1981.[5]

Maslach and colleagues defined each of these three components. Emotional exhaustion is described as the feeling of being emotionally overextended and exhausted by one's work. Exhaustion is seen by many as the key component of the burnout syndrome, and some researchers have developed alternative scoring systems to reflect this.[6,7] Exhaustion has a pervasive effect on the ability of a doctor to carry out his or her work safely and effectively. In addition, a sense of exhaustion carries over into the personal life of a burnout sufferer, affecting relationships and the ability to have a happy and fulfilling life outside of work.

The second major component, depersonalisation, is described as an unfeeling, un-empathetic and impersonal response to the interaction with patients. In effect the burnout sufferer dehumanises the person with whom they are interacting, and this leads to cold, callous behaviour and cynicism. The result is unsatisfying patient–doctor interactions, both for the doctor and the patient, which contribute to a diminished sense of personal accomplishment for the doctor, carry the potential for further stress in the form of complaints against the doctor, and result in poor health care provision for the patient.

Personal accomplishment relates to a sense of competence or achievement in one's work which results in job satisfaction or, if absent, dissatisfaction. This absence is the third major component of burnout. A poor sense of personal accomplishment has been found to be the leading feature of burnout amongst some groups of medical professionals such as physicians working in pain management in the United States.[8]

The Maslach Burnout Inventory uses a questionnaire from which a score can be given to each of these three features to identify those who are suffering from burnout and those who are at risk of burnout. This sterile, statistical way of considering a human problem is particularly useful for research, but the real-life interaction between these three components varies considerably, resulting in different degrees of distress and debilitation for sufferers.

Whilst the scope of this book is to consider the causes of burnout amongst medical professionals and specifically amongst the general practice population of the NHS, there are a number of general factors that contribute to occupational burnout in all workplaces.

In general, people are at high risk of occupational burnout when they do not feel in control of their work. It is not necessarily workload or the need to make decisions that causes stress, rather it is the lack of authority to make those decisions, otherwise known as a lack of decision latitude, which results in an inability to deal effectively with the workload, leading to unsustainable workplace stress and burnout.[9] Related to this lack of control is dysfunctional workplace dynamics, which may include workplace bullying and an unclear or ill-defined job role.

Burnout can be the product of work that is monotonous or work that is chaotic, or work that combines elements of these two apparently conflicting features.[4] Work within health care is often capable of combing these two elements, with mundane routine work frequently interspersed with complex, important and emotionally demanding tasks; perhaps this is why those working within health care find themselves at such high risk of burnout.

Low income can be a factor in the burnout, as demonstrated in a study of burnout among paediatric nurses.[10] A poor work–life balance is another contributing factor to burnout, a common imbalance that is not limited to health care professionals.[2]

Certain personality traits, such as perfectionism, competitiveness and the need to feel in control, along with habitual high achievement, put people at higher risk of burnout. These traits are common amongst medical professionals, and in fact are often selected for in those applying to medical school.

These general factors, and a host of other factors that are specific to the role of an NHS GP, can combine to create burnout which may manifest itself in a multitude of ways.

IMPACT ON THE INDIVIDUAL

As with other mental health problems, burnout can cause a wide range of psychological and physical effects. Many of these problems are also features of anxiety and depression, conditions with which burnout has an enormous degree of overlap.

Burnout has often been described as occurring in three stages, each of which may have both psychological and physical symptoms.[11] The first of these stages is known as stress arousal. This first stage is typified by difficulty concentrating, memory lapses, irritability and anxiety. Physical symptoms, like those associated with anxiety disorders, include teeth grinding, palpitations, headaches, poor sleep and loss of libido.

The second stage is the period of energy conservation during which time someone beginning to suffer with burnout will attempt to compensate for the stress they are experiencing. It is at this point that an individual's usual mechanisms for coping with stress may become overwhelmed, and so they begin to compensate in maladaptive ways. This results in avoidance behaviours including lateness, procrastination, social withdrawal and increased time off work. Avoidance behaviours can also manifest as difficulties in making decisions and problem solving which bring with them a predictable deterioration in occupational functioning. It is during this period that exhaustion can set in and psychological problems increase which may lead to self-medication and substance misuse.

The final stage is exhaustion. At this point, chronic mental health problems with anxiety and depression, including suicidality, may develop. Those experiencing this degree of burnout may increasingly rely on substance misuse as a coping strategy, so addiction may be a concomitant problem. Feelings of apathy are common and decision-making is poor, leading to poor patient care and, possibly, unethical behaviour.[12] Somatic symptoms which may also be present include non-cardiac chest pain, dizziness and chronic headaches.

It is important to recognise the features that may be present in each stage of this progression, both in ourselves and in our colleagues, but it is also important to recognise that there need not be an inexorable decline through the stages.

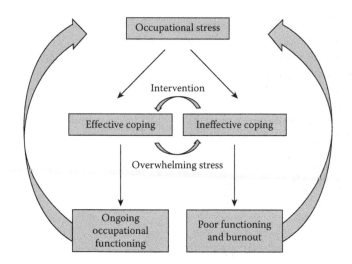

Figure 1.1 Cycle of stress and burnout.

Progression of stress and burnout can be halted and reversed if the problem is recognised and tackled (Figure 1.1).

Unfortunately, if the problem is not recognised and is left untended, there can be long-term physical and mental health consequences. Beyond chronic depressive and anxiety states, occupational stress has been linked with an increased rate of myocardial infarction, and a poor prognosis following an ischaemic event, the metabolic syndrome, and even a postulated link with the formation of stones in the urinary tract.[13–15] Burnout is very bad for your health.

Substance misuse and addiction are also strongly associated with occupational burnout. Between 10% and 15% of US physicians are thought to suffer with a substance misuse disorder, and in 1998 a British Medical Association working group found that around 1 in 15 doctors in the United Kingdom had some form of dependence on alcohol or drugs which equated to around 13,000 doctors nationally.[16,17] This can have a huge impact on professional and social functioning, and it is often a problem that is compounded by the reluctance of doctors to seek help.

Beyond the misuse of drugs and alcohol, there is also evidence that burnout can result in the development of eating disorders, including overeating, leading to overweight and obesity.[18]

The diverse symptoms of burnout can make it difficult to spot, but they ultimately combine to stop a doctor being able to function in the demanding environment of general practice. As individuals cease to work effectively, or recognise that they have a problem and opt to stop working within the NHS entirely, this has knock-on effects for the wider GP workforce who must take up the slack.

EFFECT ON THE GP WORKFORCE

In 2015 the US-based Commonwealth Fund conducted an international survey of primary care physicians based in 11 countries which included more than

1000 UK-based GPs. Amongst these NHS GPs, the survey found relatively low levels of job satisfaction and high reported levels of stress, with 59% of GPs reporting that their job was very or extremely stressful.[19] This was higher than in any other of the surveyed countries.

Levels of satisfaction were also shown to have fallen from 84% in 2012 to 67% just 3 years later. This was the steepest decline in satisfaction of any of the countries surveyed; in fact, satisfaction levels had risen in 6 of the 10 countries that were surveyed on both occasions.

In the United Kingdom, 29% of GPs reported that they intended to leave general practice within 5 years, which broke down as 17% planning to retire, 8% planning to switch careers within medicine and 4% planning to leave medicine altogether (Figure 1.2). There was a clear link between levels of perceived stress and a desire to leave general practice, with 77% of those intending to leave medicine reporting that they find their job very or extremely stressful compared to 49% of those intending to stay.[20]

On top of these worrying figures, a further 17% of GPs were unsure whether they would still be working in general practice after 5 years. Therefore, nearly half of the current workforce is either committed to leaving general practice or considering doing so in the near future.

Not only will we lose GPs from the workforce in the next 5 years, but also the Commonwealth Fund survey reported that 22% of GPs felt they had been made ill from the stress of their work within the last year; so, even amongst those GPs who intend to stay within general practice, workdays are potentially lost due to illness.

Other than those GPs nearing retirement age who may be planning to retire early, or retire as expected, a large number of GPs leaving the workforce are young. Overall, 45.5% of GP leavers between 2009 and 2014 were younger than 50, with many in the early stages of their career.[21] The loss of many of these doctors to the NHS is the gain of other countries, with a significant number each year choosing to work abroad in search of better working conditions.[22]

At a time when the government is trying to increase the overall numbers of GPs, general practice is desperately struggling to retain its existing workforce. For prospective GPs thinking of joining the specialty, this can be off-putting and whilst GP numbers increased at an average rate of 2.3% in the 10 years leading up to 2011, this rate of increase was only half that of other specialties.[23] Despite the Department of Health's intention of increasing GP trainee numbers to 3250 each year, until 2014 training numbers had stuck stubbornly below 2700 and, after the first round of recruitment for training places starting in August 2016, 30% of places remained unfilled nationally.[24,25] Currently, only 20% of medical graduates are choosing a career in general practice, well below the Department of Health's target of 50%.[26]

With recruitment suboptimal and workforce retention difficult, gaps are common in NHS general practice. For example, in 2014 the Wessex Local Medical Committees conducted a survey which found that 67% of their practices had needed to fill a vacancy in the preceding year and, of these practices, 28% had failed to recruit.[27] Numbers of GPs per 1000 head of population tend to be

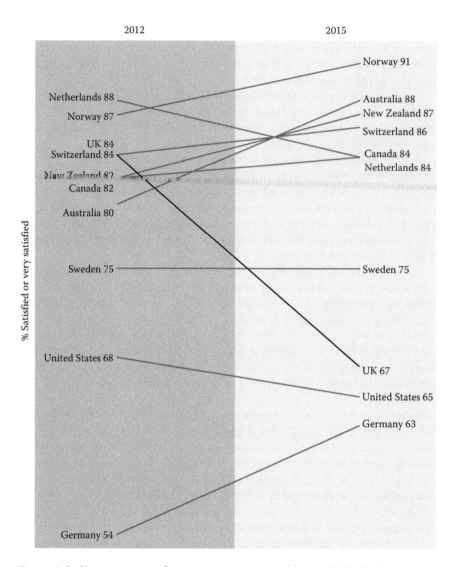

Figure 1.2 Changes in satisfaction in practicing medicine, 2012–2015. (From Davies, E., et al., *Under Pressure: What the Commonwealth Fund's 2015 International Survey of General Practitioners Means for UK General Practice*, The Health Foundation, 2016. With permission.)

lower in urban areas, in the north of England and the Midlands, which reflects particularly difficult problems with retention and recruitment in these areas.[23] These gaps in the workforce increase the workload for other GPs which then raises their risk of stress and burnout.

Despite these gloomy statistics, GPs in the United Kingdom are still providing a service that pleases their patients. In the 2015–2016 GP patient survey conducted by NHS England, 85.2% of patients rated their experience as good or very good.[28] This was however a slight decrease from that of previous years which perhaps shows how much the general practice workforce is feeling the strain and that this is now beginning to impact upon the patient experience.

The NHS is dependent on general practice, and if general practice struggles, so does the entire health care system.

EFFECT ON THE WIDER NHS

Since the creation of the NHS in 1948, general practice has been central to its structure and function. The importance of general practice to the way the NHS runs was re-iterated in 1997 when the Department of Health released 'The New NHS: Modern, Dependable' and more recently in 2014's 'NHS Five Year Forward View' which outlined plans to move more services into the community, away from secondary care.[29,30]

With GPs providing the vast bulk of patient contacts, and the vast bulk of patient care, and with their role coordinating the care provided by increasingly fragmented secondary care providers, the centrality of general practice to the NHS is obvious to those who use it and to those who run it. It is for this reason that as long as there is a will to have an NHS, general practice must ultimately be supported and guided through each of its crises.

A GP workforce struggling with stress and burnout, working ineffectively and providing poor patient care is self-evidently bad for the system, and the system is already demonstrably beginning to suffer because of this. Tackling GP stress and burnout should therefore be central to any strategy to improving NHS services.

Poor primary care practice, or an overwhelmed primary care service, shifts the burden of its work towards secondary care, either by higher rates of routine referrals or by causing increased attendance to emergency departments.

Increased attendance at the accident & emergency department (A&E) creates a rising number of breaches of the government's 4-h A&E target and an increased number of admissions to hospital beds (Figure 1.3).

In response to this problem, NHS England launched the 'Avoiding Unplanned Admissions' enhanced service in 2015 as an attempt to reduce the number of emergency admissions amongst people at high risk of hospital admission by asking GPs to create care plans for them. The intention was to ease the burden on secondary care but, from the viewpoint of a beleaguered primary care workforce, the strategy was backward, adding an extra burden to a general practice work-force that was already struggling with its workload.

Furthermore, despite the enhanced service, the waiting time targets for A&E, which is the government's chosen metric for measuring A&E success, were not met for any month except July in the year 2015–2016 and, in the quarter covering October–December 2015, breaches of the 4-h wait were at their highest level in more than a decade.[31]

Clearly, the causes for this were multifactorial and included problems of staff retention and recruitment within emergency medicine, and difficulty discharging

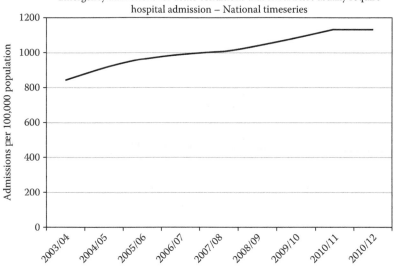

Figure 1.3 Rise in emergency admissions. (Courtesy of NHS England Analytical Service, *Improving General Practice – A Call to Action, Evidence Pack*. 2014.)

patients at the end of their hospital admissions due to problems providing social care, but difficulty accessing GP services were amongst the relevant issues.

A survey conducted by the Royal College of Emergency Medicine suggested that 15% of A&E attenders could have been treated in the community. Moreover, data from the GP Patient Survey show that the number of people able to get timely appointments with their GPs had fallen from 88% in 2011 to 85% in 2016 and, of those unable to get a convenient GP appointment, around 4% attended A&E instead.[31]

The pressures contributing to GP burnout, which will be discussed in detail in Chapters 2 and 3, clearly impact the rest of the NHS. A system built around primary care needs to have primary care providers who are supported to work at their optimum.

CONCLUSION

Burnout is a common phenomenon that has an increasingly deleterious effect on GPs, the wider NHS and, ultimately, patients. The problem leads to a vicious cycle; burnt-out GPs leave practice which increases the pressures on the rest of the workforce who are subsequently at higher risk of burning out.

This is already an urgent issue and, with nearly half the workforce considering leaving general practice within the next 5 years, we may merely be at the edge of the precipice with the possibility of things getting very much worse without immediate action.

REFERENCES

1. Freudenberger HJ. Staff burnout. *J Soc Issues.* 1974;30(1):159–65.
2. Hammig O, Bauer GF. Work, work-life conflict and health in an industrial work environment. *Occup Med (Lond).* 2014;64(1):34–8. doi: 10.1093/occmed/kqt127.
3. Mateen FJ, Dorji C. Health-care worker burnout and the mental health imperative. *Lancet.* 2009;374(9690):595–7.
4. Tidy, C. Occupational Burnout. *Patient.co.uk.* 2015. http://patient.info/doctor/occupational-burnout. Accessed on 19 July, 2017.
5. Maslach C, Jackson SE. *MBI: Maslach Burnout Inventory.* Manual Research Edition. Palo Alto, CA: Consulting Psychologists Press; 1986.
6. Gómez-Urquiza JL, Monsalve-Reyes CS, San Luis-Costas C, Fernández-Castillo R, Aguayo-Estremera R, Cañadas-de la Fuente GA. Risk factors and burnout levels in primary care nurses: A systematic review. *Aten Primaria.* 2017;49(2):77–85.
7. Kristensen TS, Borritz M, Villadsen E, Christensen KB. The Copenhagen Burnout Inventory: A new tool for the assessment of burnout. *Work Stress.* 2005;19(3):192–207.
8. Kroll HR, Macaulay T, Jesse M. A preliminary survey examining predictors of burnout in pain medicine physicians in the United States. *Pain Physician.* 2016;19(5):E689–96.
9. Wong CA, Spence Laschinger HK. The influence of frontline manager job strain on burnout, commitment and turnover intention: A cross-sectional study. *Int J Nurs Stud.* 2015;52(12):1824–33.
10. Akman O, Ozturk C, Bektas M, Ayar D, Armstrong MA. Job satisfaction and burnout among paediatric nurses. *J Nurs Manag.* 2016;24(7):923–33.
11. Kumar, S. Burnout and Doctors: Prevalence, Prevention and Intervention. *Healthcare.* 2016;4(3):37.
12. Everall R, Paulson, B. Burnout and Secondary Traumatic Stress: Impact on Ethical Behaviour. *Canadian Journal of Counselling.* 2004;38(1):25–35.
13. Consoli SM. Occupational stress and myocardial infarction. *Presse Med.* 2015;44(7–8):745–51.
14. Almadi T, Cathers I, Chow CM. Associations among work-related stress, cortisol, inflammation, and metabolic syndrome. *Psychophysiology.* 2013;50(9):821–30.
15. Arzoz-Fabregas M, Ibarz-Servio L, Edo-Izquierdo S, Doladé-Botías M, Fernandez-Castro J, Roca-Antonio J. Chronic stress and calcium oxalate stone disease: Is it a potential recurrence risk factor? *Urolithiasis.* 2013;41(2):119–27.
16. Oreskovich MR, Kaups KL, Balch CM, et al. Prevalence of alcohol use disorders among American surgeons. *Arch Surg.* 2012;147:168–74.
17. Sick Doctors Trust. Overview of Addiction. http://sick-doctors-trust.co.uk/page/addiction. Accessed on 19 July, 2017.

18. Nevanpera NJ, Hopsu L, Kuosma E, et al. Occupational burnout, eating behavior, and weight among working women. *Am J Clin Nutr.* 2012;95(4):934–43.

19. The Commonwealth Fund. 2015 Commonwealth Fund International Survey of Primary Care Physicians in 10 Nations. http://www.commonwealthfund. org/interactives-and-data/surveys/2015/2015-international-survey. Accessed on 19 July, 2017.

20. Davies E, Martin S, Gershlick B. *Under pressure: What the Commonwealth Fund's 2015 International Survey of General Practitioners means for the UK.* 2016. http://www.health.org.uk/publication/ underpressure#sthash.3qqLghqH.dput. Accessed on 19 July, 2017.

21. Health & Social Care Information Centre. *General and Personal Medical Services, England—2004–2014, as at 30 September.* http://www.hscic. gov.uk/catalogue/PUB16934. Accessed on 19 July, 2017.

22. Davies, M. GP Brain Drain is a 'Signifcant Danger' Says BMA. *Pulse.* 2016. http://www.pulsetoday.co.uk/home/finance-and-practice-life-news/ gpbrain-drain-is-a-significant-danger-says-bma/20003804.fullarticle. Accessed on 19 July, 2017.

23. NHS England Analytical Service. *Improving General Practice – A Call to Action. Evidence Pack.* 2014. http://www.england.nhs.uk/wp-content/ uploads/2013/09/igp-cta-evid.pdf. Accessed on 19 July, 2017.

24. GP Taskforce. *Securing the Future GP Workforce: Delivering the Mandate on GP Expansion.* GP Taskforce final report. Leeds: Health Education England; 2014.

25. Kaffash, J. 30% of GP Training Places Remain Unfilled. *Pulse.* 2016. http:// www.pulsetoday.co.uk/your-practice/practice-topics/education/30-of- gp-training-places-remain-unfilled/20031494.fullarticle. Accessed on 19 July, 2017.

26. Lambert T, Goldacre M. Trends in doctors' early career choices for general practice in the UK: Longitudinal questionnaire surveys. *Br J Gen Pract.* 2011;61:e397–403.

27. Wessex, LMC. GP Recruitment Crisis. *Press Release.* 2014. https://www. wessexlmcs.com/gprecruitmentcrisis. Accessed on 19 July, 2017.

28. NHS England. *GP Patient Survey 2015–16.* 2016. https://www.england. nhs.uk/statistics/2016/07/07/gp-patient-survey-2015-16/. Accessed on 19 July, 2017.

29. Department of Health. *The New NHS: Modern, Dependable.* Department of Health; 1997. www.gov.uk/government/uploads/system/uploads/ attachment_data/file/266003/newnhs.pdf. Accessed on 19 July, 2017.

30. NHS England. *NHS Five Year Forward View.* NHS England; 2014. www.england.nhs.uk/ourwork/futurenhs/. Accessed on 19 July, 2017.

31. King's Fund. *What's Going on in A&E? The Key Questions Answered.* http://www.kingsfund.org.uk/projects/urgent-emergency-care/urgent- and-emergency-care-mythbusters. Accessed on 19 July, 2017.

2

External pressures

DR. ADAM STATEN
The Red House Surgery, Bletchley, UK

There are few who would deny that being a doctor is an inherently stressful job. It is intellectually demanding and involves complex decision making and, on top of this, there is an emotional component to almost all that we do. We frequently deal with people who are frightened, unhappy or angry and with people who may make us feel frightened, unhappy or angry.

It would be impossible to remove all the stress from our work and many doctors would not consider it desirable to do so because it is our involvement with these intellectually, emotionally and psychologically challenging patients that also provides so much of the satisfaction in our work.

But there is more to being a doctor than just seeing patients. Doctors do not work in isolation and cannot simply work in a way of their choosing. Instead, they form a professional body that requires both internal and external validation, and they work within health care systems to which they must conform. In particular, doctors working within a state-funded health care system such as the National Health Service (NHS) have heavy regulatory demands put upon them because they must justify to the tax-paying patient that they are performing to an appropriate standard and working in an appropriate way.

As both our patients and the government seek to make us more accountable, more transparent, and, perhaps above all, more cost effective, a wide range of external pressures have been put upon general practitioners (GPs) working within the NHS, and this has added a burden of administration, time consumption, financial cost, and litigation on top of the pressures inherent to the job of caring for patients.

In the National GP Worklife Survey conducted by the University of Manchester in 2015, GPs cited meeting the requirements of external bodies as the second biggest stressor in their job after increasing workload.[1] Many doctors feel the external pressures of regulatory bodies and the continual organisational changes that seem to typify life in the NHS have fundamentally altered their ability to practice in the way that they wish.[2] So, whilst the stress of dealing with patients can lead to professional satisfaction, the stress of dealing with external pressures tends to lead to a lack of job satisfaction, a key feature of burnout.

THE QUALITY OUTCOMES FRAMEWORK

The Quality Outcomes Framework (QOF) was introduced to the GP contract in 2004 and was, at the time, the largest health-related pay-for-performance scheme in the world. The intention was to raise the standard of care for chronic illnesses in primary care by incentivising GPs to hit targets in several 'quality indicators'. It was, theoretically at least, a voluntary scheme, but with up to 25% of a GP's salary linked to the QOF, few GP practices opted out of the scheme.

There seemed to be some initial successes, particularly in reducing health inequalities around the country, and the scheme proved surprisingly popular amongst GPs who found the initial targets easy to meet as a result of governmental underestimation of the baseline quality of care in general practice.[3]

The QOF evolved over time and the shifting goalposts of the annually set quality indicators left GPs feeling largely disillusioned and disengaged with a scheme that increasingly seemed to be a cynical political tool to curb GP pay. Quality indicators often seemed to achieve marginal gain but demanded a high workload, and they seemed set to meet managerial and political agenda rather than clinical need.[4]

The narrow targets, based on single diseases, were shown to be of no benefit in the multi-morbid patients that are the reality of daily practice, nor did they reduce mortality in cancer, ischaemic heart disease, or all non-targeted conditions.[5,6] Moreover, QOF indicators, and the remuneration attached to them, were shown to be poorly targeted to achieve maximum gain.[7]

There was a widespread feeling that valuable consultation time was taken up with QOF-related tasks. This created a clash between what GPs felt they needed to do to deliver proper patient care and what they pragmatically had to do to ensure that they got paid and to ensure that adequate funds continued to flow into the surgery. Naturally, this left many doctors feeling dissatisfied with the way in which they were practicing. The QOF is now being steadily dismantled but will undoubtedly be replaced with another scheme and we must guard against this intrusion into clinical practice occurring again.

THE CARE QUALITY COMMISSION

The Care Quality Commission (CQC), created in 2009, has also been blamed for increasing rates of burnout. GP surgeries are currently inspected every 5 years and meeting the requirements of a CQC inspection imposes an enormous administrative burden on practices which must provide paper trails detailing all manner of clinical and non-clinical activities, as well as producing policies on everything from child safeguarding to handling complaints. To date, 4% of practices have been found to be inadequate according to the CQC's standards.

The move toward increased inspection, assessment and regulation is a global phenomenon and is causing discontent amongst doctors internationally because of the atmosphere of mistrust it creates and the extra burden it places on medical professionals.[8,9] In the United Kingdom the burden of assessment and inspection is the highest in Europe.[10] The CQC has been criticised by doctors for creating a culture of fear with its intensive inspections being punitive rather than serving the stated purpose of driving quality improvement.[10]

The CQC has also been criticised for its working practices which include a perpetually backlogged schedule of inspections and long delays between inspections and the production of reports during which time the fate of GP practices, which can include closure, is left hanging.[11] At a governmental level the CQC has faced repeated and persistent concerns that it is not fit for purpose.[12]

POLITICAL MANDATE AND CONTINUAL STRUCTURAL REFORM

Both the QOF and the CQC have been politically driven initiatives and are symptomatic of political interference in health care. Over the last three decades, there have been a total of 15 major structural reforms of the NHS.[13] Many of these reforms have been cyclical, with new governments dusting off the forgotten and failed reforms of previous governments, and the implementation of change is often so rapid that it occurs before any formal legislation has been put in place, with the nuts and bolts of reorganisation being worked out without great thought or preparation.[13]

There is little evidence that structural reforms of any kind are of benefit but, in any case, these reforms are seldom retrospectively analysed to assess why they did not work.[13] However, this was not the case with perhaps the most notorious of these major reforms, those that were introduced by the Health Secretary Andrew Lansley in 2010. Described by fellow conservatives as 'unintelligible gobbledygook', and considered by many to be the biggest mistake of the coalition government,[14] these reforms were introduced at breakneck speed and were so ill considered and cack-handedly implemented that the King's Fund almost immediately commissioned a report into what had gone wrong entitled 'Never Again?'.[15]

These reforms, as is often the case, were billed as a means of cutting bureaucracy and saving money but in fact involved the dismantlement of 162 organisations and the creation of between 500 and 600 new organisations. The government optimistically estimated that the cost of the reforms was around £1.5 billion, but many think this a wild underestimate.[16]

Extreme though these reforms may have been, they were not atypical. Every reform comes with a financial and administrative cost and leaves those involved with actually providing patient care dizzied and bemused. No sooner have newly formed organisations got to grip with their role and finally started to function, then another reform leaves GPs and other health professionals scrambling to learn the nature of, and learn how to engage with, a whole glut of new organisations, all whilst attempting to maintain patient care.

There is also continual, lower level political interference with all aspects of health care provision. An example of this was the politically driven initiative of the dementia-enhanced service, designed to improve dementia diagnosis rates, which was imposed in the 2013–2014 GP contract despite opposition from the Royal College.

Similarly, the NHS 'Health Check' was launched in 2009 by the government to prevent vascular disease despite a lack of robust evidence to support its implementation. It has been continued despite subsequent evidence demonstrating poor uptake by patients and its failure to identify those most at risk of heart disease, presumably because it is politically expedient to demonstrate activity in this area of public concern.[17]

There is a tension at the heart of the NHS. As it is funded by the tax payer, there is a feeling that politicians must remain ultimately accountable for the service, but this leaves it at the mercy of a carousel of political strategists who plan only for the next election cycle. This creates an environment of tremendous uncertainty for NHS employees and a sensation that health care provision is beyond the control of those who must provide it, robbing them of 'decision latitude'. These two factors contribute hugely to occupational stress and burnout.

A NEGATIVE MEDIA PORTRAYAL

In a study investigating the reasons why GPs leave the NHS, 63.4% of GPs surveyed cited a negative media image as a contributory factor.[2] As a result of headlines such as 'These Overpaid GPs Must Stop Whingeing' (*The Times*, 28 May, 2014), it has entered the public consciousness that GPs are overpaid, underworked and whining. The continual denigration of the work that GPs do is incredibly demoralising and, to some, this lack of appreciation feels like a betrayal of the old-fashioned doctor–patient relationship in which the doctor's professional role is valued and respected. Not only does this erode the sense of personal accomplishment for the job that GPs do, but the sensation of being at odds with the public that they serve can contribute to the experience of depersonalisation which can lead to a lack of compassion and callous, disinterested treatment.

In a world in which the media feed operates 24 h a day, and appears on ubiquitous platforms from the TV in our front room to the phone in our pocket, a continual negative portrayal can feel smothering. The pervasive and pernicious media coverage of health issues and health professionals is a significant contributory factor to GP stress.

A MORE LITIGIOUS SOCIETY

Despite medical care running at its highest standard ever, rates of malpractice claims continue to escalate, with a rate of 'claims inflation' running at around 10% per year.[18] Currently the NHS litigation authority, which deals with negligence claims against NHS bodies, sets aside around £26 billion each year, or approximately one quarter the value of the NHS budget, to deal with malpractice suits and in the year 2015–2016 it paid out nearly £1 billion in damages to patients.[19] The rise in costs has been attributed to, amongst other factors, more claims being made because the NHS is more busy, more incidents being reported and a higher proportion of these incidents resulting in claims, and disproportionately high claimant legal fees (Figure 2.1).[19]

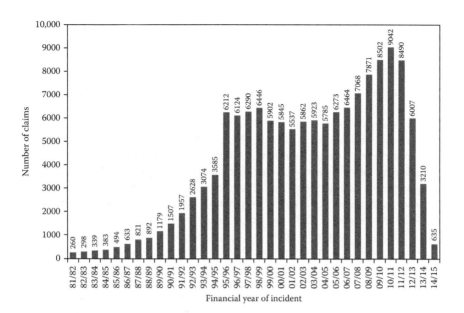

Figure 2.1 Number of Claims Processed by the NHS Litigation Authority According to Financial Year of Incident (correct at 31 May 2015). (From: NHS Litigation Authority, Factsheet 3: Information on claims 2015–2016.)

The average GP can now expect to be sued twice in a 35-year career, and this is particularly problematic for GPs because they do not benefit from the funds and protection of the NHS Litigation Authority and who, unlike their secondary care colleagues, do not have crown indemnity.[18] So, as the cost of litigation rises, GPs have seen the cost of their personal medical indemnity spiral. In 2016 a survey of GPs by *GPOnline* found that 93% had seen the cost of their indemnity rise in the last year, and 53% of full-time GPs were paying more than £7500 to be indemnified annually.[20]

Beyond the financial cost, the psychological cost of the current legal environment can be disastrous. This process can, of course, result in prolonged periods of stress resulting in the emotional and psychological exhaustion typical of burnout, but it can also cause serious mental ill health in the form of depression and suicidality. Between 2005 and 2013, 24 doctors committed suicide whilst under investigation by the General Medical Council (GMC), with a further four suspected suicides.[21] Taking GMC referrals as a proxy for other kinds of complaint, it is clear that the psychological impact on doctors of a more litigious society is not to be ignored.

CONCLUSION

Stress in the world of medicine is inevitable but there are many features of life in NHS general practice that make it more stressful than perhaps it need be. To an extent it is also inevitable that GPs working within the system will be subject to

I HAVE ALWAYS BEEN A WORKAHOLIC

Dr. Zoe Norris

GP Blogger and UK Chair of GPC Sessional Subcommittee

I have always been a workaholic. That has been my coping mechanism. If it's busy, work harder. A GP down? Just work harder. More patients than appointments? If I work harder, that will solve it. That got me through my medical training, my junior doctor years, my time as a salaried GP, and was my approach as a partner. Then I found myself in a position where working harder wasn't working. I was putting in way over my hours, arriving at work at 7.30 am, leaving at 10.30 pm. I didn't stop to eat or drink. I never said no to a request. I thought if I could just keep going it would be fine. I stopped sleeping, waking in the night lying there thinking about work. I was drinking too much to try and relax. I lived off takeaways, too tired to cook. I was tired all the time, aching all over. I diagnosed myself with a million weird and wonderful conditions but never had time to see my own GP. I stopped caring about my patients – every name on the list of appointments was another barrier. Another mountain to climb before I could stop putting on this face of a friendly competent doctor, and turn my attention to the mountains of paperwork waiting for me. Every extra name that needed a home visit, or a phone call – I resented them all. My notes were too brief, my attention span short. I ordered test after test because I couldn't think clearly or trust my own judgement. I knew I wasn't doing a good job but I could only think it was because I wasn't trying hard enough. I stopped caring. I turned into the kind of GP I had always scorned – impersonal, impatient, unfeeling. When I became hysterical while on the phone to a hospital nurse one night who I was trying to discuss a patient with, I suddenly realised I couldn't carry on like this. I went home that night ready to look for another career, and leave medicine. I was 34 years old.

external stressors of the kind described above, but this does not mean that they must be accepted without protest. The aims of projects such as the QOF and the CQC are, at heart, laudable even if their implementation and execution have been imperfect. In situations such as this, it is the duty of GPs to voice concern, resist when necessary and be flexible when appropriate because there are mechanisms available by which GPs can improve the system.

REFERENCES

1. Gibson J, Checkland K, Coleman A, Hann M, Mccall R, Spooner S, Sutton M. *Eighth National GP Worklife Survey.* Policy Research Unit in Commissioning and the Healthcare System (PRUComm), 2015.

2. Doran N, Fox F, Rodham K, Taylor G, Harris M. Lost to the NHS: A mixed methods study of why GPs leave practice early in England. *Br J Gen Pract* 2016;66(643):e128–35.

3. Doran T, Fullwood C, Kontopantelis E, Reeves D. Effect of financial incentives on inequalities in the delivery of primary clinical care in England: Analysis of clinical activity indicators for the quality and outcomes framework. *Lancet* 2008;372(9640):728–36.

4. Roland and Guthrie. Quality and Outcomes Framework: What have we learnt? *BMJ* 2016;354:i4060.

5. Ruscitto A, Mercer SW, Morales D, Guthrie B. Accounting for multimorbidity in pay for performance: A modelling study using UK Quality and Outcomes Framework data. *Br J Gen Pract* 2016;66(649):e561–7.

6. Ryan AM, Krinsky S, Kontopantelis E, Doran T. Long-term evidence for the effect of pay-for-performance in primary care on mortality in the UK: A population study. *Lancet* 2016;388:268–74.

7. Fleetcroft R, Steel N, Cookson R, Walker S, Howe A. Incentive payments are not related to expected health gain in the pay for performance scheme for UK primary care: Cross-sectional analysis. *BMC Health Serv Res* 2012;12:94.

8. Grimsgaand C. *Mistroens pris [The price of mistrust]*. Dagens Medisin, 17 November 2015. www.dagensmedisin.no/artikler/2015/11/17/mistroens-pris. (In Norwegian.). Accessed on 22 July, 2017.

9. Wachter, R. How Measurement Fails Doctors and Teachers. *New York Times*. 2016. http://www.nytimes.com/2016/01/17/opinion/sunday/how-measurementfails-doctors-and-teachers.html?_r=0. Accessed on 22 July, 2017.

10. McCarthy M. Too much scrutiny is bad for general practice. *BMJ* 2016;353:i2151.

11. Kmietowicz Z. Care Quality Commission is still not up to the job, MPs' report finds. *BMJ* 2015;351:h6744.

12. House of Commons Committee of Public Accounts. *Care Quality Commission. Twelfth report of session* 2015–16. 2015. www.publications.parliament.uk/pa/cm201516/cmselect/cmpubacc/501/501.pdf. Accessed on 22 July, 2017.

13. Walshe K. Reorganisation of the NHS in England. *BMJ* 2010;341:c3843.

14. Chorley M. "Unintelligible gobbledygook" of NHS reforms were our biggest mistake in government, senior Tories admit. *Daily Mail*, 13 October 2014. www.dailymail.co.uk/news/article-2790785/unintelligible-gobbledygook-nhs-reforms-biggest-mistake-government-senior-tories-admit.html

15. King's Fund. *Never Again? The Story of the Health and Social Care Act 2012*. 2012. The King's Fund: London.

16. Walshe K. Counting the cost of England's NHS reorganisation. *BMJ* 2014;349:g6340.

17. Price, C. RCGP urges halt to NHS Health Checks until 'robust evidence' exists. *Pulse*. 2015. http://www.pulsetoday.co.uk/clinical/cardiovascular/rcgp-urges-halt-tonhs-health-checks-until-robust-evidence-exists/20009964.fullarticle. Accessed on 22 July, 2017.
18. Bower, E. Why are medical indemnity fees rising? *GP Online*. 2015. http://www.gponline.com/why-medical-indemnity-fees-rising/article/1358134. Accessed on 22 July, 2017.
19. NHS Litigation Authority. NHS Litigation authority reports and accounts 2015/16. 2016. NHSLA: London. http://www.nhsla.com/AboutUs/Documents/NHS_Litigation_Authority_Annual_Report_and_Accounts_2015-2016.pdf. Accessed on 22 July, 2017.
20. Millett, D. Exclusive: Rise in medical indemnity costs accelerates as 90% of GPs face higher fees. *Pulse*. 2016. http://www.gponline.com/exclusive-rise-medical-indemnity- accelerates-90-gps-face-higher-fees/article/1401723. Accessed on 22 July, 2017.
21. GMC. Doctors who commit suicide while under GMC fitness to practise investigation. General Medical Council: London. 2014.

3

Pressures of the job

DR. ADAM STATEN
The Red House Surgery, Bletchley, UK

The clinical pressures of general practice are dynamic. Because general practitioners (GPs) are embedded in the communities in which they work, the nature of their work changes rapidly with the population around them. The human geography of the United Kingdom has changed dramatically in the past 60 years, and it is continuing to change. These shifting demographics place new demands on the medical profession.

The world of medicine is also continually changing, and our ability to investigate, diagnose and treat illness has changed beyond recognition from as recently as 20 or 30 years ago. This means there is more for GPs to do for each patient and more to squeeze into each consultation. It also means that patients expect more from their doctors.

Despite the changing nature of the population and the advances in medical science, GPs continue to work in a way that is broadly recognisable to the way in which they worked when the National Health Service (NHS) was founded. So, there is friction between what is expected of GPs and what they can deliver. This increases the inherent pressures of the job, so contributing to increased stress and burnout.

INCREASING WORKLOAD

The population of the United Kingdom is growing, and it is a population that has become used to free access to doctors over several generations. With the increasing ability of modern medicine to make people better, and to prevent them getting ill, there is now more reason than ever for people to visit their GP. These factors are reflected in the year-on-year increase in the number of GP consultations that are undertaken each year, a number which has been steadily increasing since the mid-1990s. In 2008, GPs performed around 300 million consultations, and it is now thought that the figure is more than 340 million (Figure 3.1).[1]

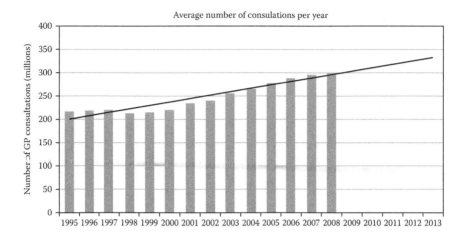

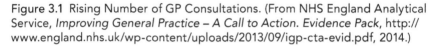

Figure 3.1 Rising Number of GP Consultations. (From NHS England Analytical Service, *Improving General Practice – A Call to Action. Evidence Pack*, http:// www.england.nhs.uk/wp-content/uploads/2013/09/igp-cta-evid.pdf, 2014.)

A recent analysis of 100 million UK GP consultations found that not only are raw numbers of consultations increasing, but consultations are getting longer, probably reflecting the more complex nature of the workload. This study found that the average number of consultations per person each year had risen by just over 10% in the 6 years between 2008 and 2014, with the average person now seeing their GP over five times each year. The number of telephone consultations had doubled over the same period and the number of face-to-face consultations had risen by more than 5%. Overall, the clinical workload was thought to have increased by around 16%.[2] The authors also noted that they had not taken into account the workload associated with administration or management which, as already discussed (see Chapter 2), has also increased significantly in recent years.

Increasing workload was cited as the top stressor by the GPs surveyed in the National GP Worklife Survey in 2015,[3] and the changing and growing nature of the general practice workload, and the associated stress of this change and growth, emerged as the main theme in a study looking at the retention of the general practice workforce.[4] Similarly, a survey of GPs who had retried early, or who were planning to do so, found that the increasing workload was a key factor in making their decision,[5] demonstrating that the workload is having a direct impact on the NHS' ability to retain GPs.

The causes for this increase in workload are multifactorial and complex, but it is clear that managing this workload effectively at an individual and a systemic level is key, both to avoiding GP burnout and to maintaining and growing the strength of the GP workforce.

A POPULATION INCREASING IN AGE AND MORBIDITY

The population of the United Kingdom is not just growing in size; as with other developed nations, the population is aging. Life expectancy continues to rise such that girls born in 2012 can expect to live to 83 years old, compared to 49 in 1901, and by 2032 female life expectancy at birth may be as high as 87 years (Figure 3.2).[6]

The growth in the population will not be evenly spread across the age groups. Over the next 20 years, the population aged between 15–64 years will increase by 7%, but the population of over-85s will increase by 106%.[6]

This older population will bring with it a burden of morbidity. Currently, just over half of the population identify themselves as having a long-term health complaint,[1] but predictably, long-term conditions are more common amongst the elderly, with 58% of those over 60 complaining of a long-term health problem compared to 14% of those under 40.[7] This is reflected in the fact that whilst rates of GP consultations are increasing across the age ranges, the most significant increase in consultation rates is amongst older people.[1]

Whilst recorded prevalence is increasing for the majority of diseases, what is arguably most challenging for GPs is the rise in multi-morbidity, and multi-morbidity is rising rapidly.[1] By 2018, the number of people living with three or more long-term conditions is expected to be more than 2.9 million which equates to between 4% and 5% of the total population.[6]

Standing at the heart of health care, GPs are the lynch pin of care provision for these complex patients and are likely to shoulder the greatest load in dealing with this issue.

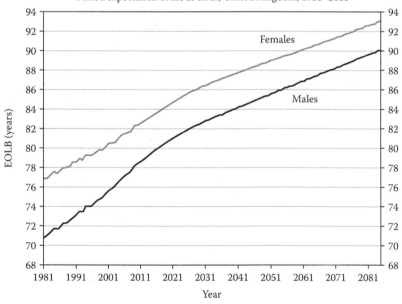

Period expectation of life at birth, United Kingdom, 1981–2085

Figure 3.2 Rising Life Expectancy over the Coming Years. (From Office for National Statistics, *Mortality Assumptions, 2010-Based National Population Projections*, http://webarchive.nationalarchives.gov.uk/20160105160709/http://www.ons.gov.uk/ons/dcp171776_237747.pdf, 2011.)

SQUEEZED BUDGETS

NHS general practice offers fantastic value for money. With less than 9% of the total NHS budget allocated to primary care in recent years, GPs have been able to provide 90% of patient contacts.[8] Perhaps it has been the ability of GPs to squeeze the pennies and still deliver high-quality care that has enabled governments to consistently overlook general practice funding so that, despite the growing pressures on primary care, funding has remained relatively static.[1]

Because of this discrepancy between funding and demand, a funding gap has begun to open up which could become as large as £2.7 billion annually by the 2020–2021 fiscal year. A poll conducted for the Royal College of General Practitioners in 2013 found that 81% of GPs no longer feel that they have adequate funding to continue to provide high-quality patient care.[8]

Between 2005 and 2006 and 2012 and 2013, expenses for GP practices rose from 55.1% to 62.5% of partners' gross earnings, resulting in a real terms drop of partner income of almost a quarter.[9] As practices have struggled to remain profitable, the income of salaried GPs has also been severely squeezed. This has made salaried posts less attractive with the knock-on effect that many GPs have found locuming to be more lucrative than taking a salaried post, and this has added to the recruitment woes of many practices.

This potentially traps practices in a vicious cycle of expense. Unable to offer an attractive salary and recruit permanent staff, practices are forced to the extra expense of locums which eats up yet more of the practice budget. Unchecked, this has the potential to undermine the entire independent contractor model of general practice by rendering it financially unsustainable.

For many doctors, and for many surgeries, these financial difficulties have been too much. A poll in 2016 conducted by the British Medical Association revealed that 1 in 10 practices consider themselves financially unsustainable and that more than 500 practices were forced to close between 2009 and 2014.[10,11]

In recent years, many GPs have found themselves working harder and feeling less rewarded. With regard to burnout, this is a toxic mixture of occupational stress and lack of job satisfaction, and the financial struggle, and the uncertainty that this brings, has been a major factor in the current workforce crisis.

TIME PRESSURES

The 10-min appointment was specified as the minimum appointment length in the 2004 GP contract, but it was widely adopted as the standard appointment length as it was generally felt to be the longest appointment that could be offered with a realistic prospect of meeting demand. But with the increasing pressures of general practice, both those inherent to an ageing and multi-morbid population and those imposed upon GPs by outside agencies, the 10-min appointment is beginning to burst at the seams.

The analysis of 100 million consultations demonstrated that whilst GPs are offering 10-min appointments on paper, the actual time spent with each patient is steadily increasing.[2] As the clinical and administrative workload of each consultation increases, the time allocated to other tasks gets squeezed so that GPs struggle to make the adequate notes needed to ensure good continuity of care and protect themselves from litigation. Indeed, GPs struggle to form the personal relationships with their patients that have until now been such a rewarding aspect of the job.

The 10-min appointment can be both unsatisfying and potentially dangerous, and it is becoming an increasing source of stress for UK GPs. Around 92% of GPs report spending less than 15 min with each patient and, in this respect, the United Kingdom is a significant outlier in comparison to the other countries surveyed in the Commonwealth Fund survey. Only 29% of GPs from other countries reported spending less than 15 min per patient.[12] In the United Kingdom, just 26% of GPs are satisfied with the amount of time they spend with patients compared to 59% in other countries.[12]

UK GPs find themselves between a rock and a hard place. There is an incessant drive for rapid access to appointments, but rapid access requires a high volume of appointments which can only be delivered by shortening their length. These shorter appointments make it difficult to deliver high-quality care, and GPs are then criticised for this. It feels unwinnable.

As a response to these time constraints, it is common for surgeries to request that their patients bring only one problem to each appointment. This could be seen as a systemic example of an ineffective coping mechanism being, as it is, a form of sanctioned procrastination, pushing today's problems into the future and requiring patients to use up yet more valuable appointments. As discussed in Chapter 1, ineffective coping mechanisms are a sign of impending burnout. It is clear that there must be change. Careful consideration must be given to what we prioritise: patient access or patient care.

INCREASING DEPENDENCE OF PATIENTS ON DOCTORS

In 2015, the GP support group *Resilient GP* surveyed a group of GPs for their most 'inappropriate' requests from patients. The list included requests for a GP to perform a home visit to change batteries in a TV remote control and a request for surgery because a patient's chin looked too fat on Facebook. At the time this was hailed by many to demonstrate the contemptuous use patients make of general practice and the enormous amount of time wasted on inappropriate tasks. However, seen in another light, this could be taken as a demonstration of how dependent patients have become on their family doctors. Not only do they seek help from their GPs for their medical problems, but they seek help and advice from their GPs on any and all problems.

In the United Kingdom, several generations have now readily been able to seek the advice of a medical professional, and this has eroded the traditional reliance on support networks, such as grandparents, who offered common-sense medical advice on minor medical ailments when doctors were not so accessible. This is compounded by the fragmentation of traditional support networks as lives have become more mobile. Many people simply do not have the support networks around them from whom to ask advice.

Whatever your view may be on the use of GP appointments for reasons such as those detailed in the *Resilient GP* survey, there is no doubt that this increased reliance on GPs as a source of social as well as medical support is an extra burden to primary care. It is a burden that frustrates some doctors who feel that their job satisfaction is diminished by such requests. This is particularly so if the doctor is already suffering from a degree of depersonalisation which leads to a reduced sense of empathy for patients whose requests for help may simply be a sign of isolation.

RISING PATIENT EXPECTATIONS

The doctor–patient relationship has changed dramatically in recent decades. Gone are the days of deference and blind faith from patients. Now the relationship has crept much closer to service provision, almost a provider–customer relationship, with patients expecting from their doctors not only good medical treatment but also openness, honesty and a respectful and courteous manner.

Our patients are also better informed than ever before with Internet access granting them the ability to read research and opinion as never before. They therefore often attend the surgery forearmed with an expectation of what their condition is, who should be treating it and how it should be treated.

A General Medical Council (GMC) survey found that all of these factors were amongst the reasons for the 100% rise in complaints it had received between 2007 and 2012.[13] These rising expectations have been playing on the minds of GPs in the United Kingdom for many years. For example, a study of GP principals leaving UK practice back in 2002 found that rising patient expectations, and the extra workload resulting from them, influenced many of their decisions to quit.[14]

Few would argue that patients should not have the right to expect openness, honesty and treatment with respect, but the difficulty with high patient expectation comes when the expectation cannot be met by a resource limited system such as the NHS. This puts the GP in a position of confounding expectations which, if not done well, can distress or anger the patient and damage the therapeutic relationship. Explaining why you are failing to meet a patient's expectations needs to be done sensitively and this is not easy, particularly within the constraints of a general practice appointment. Herein lies a major problem as some studies have shown that up to 70% of medical litigation results from such failures in communication.[15]

It is not wrong that patients have high expectations; indeed, expectations amongst patients should rise as the capabilities of modern medicine increase. Managing these expectations however is increasingly difficult in the pressured environment of general practice and this brings its own, extra stress with it.

POOR COORDINATION BETWEEN PRIMARY AND SECONDARY CARE

The NHS had division between primary care and secondary care woven into its fabric from its inception, but this division was formalised, and arguably entrenched, by the formation of the internal market and the purchaser–provider split in 1991. This divided the medical community not only along the lines of those who cared for patients in hospital and those who cared for them in the community but also put them on opposite sides of the negotiating table.

As care in various specialities has coalesced into tertiary and quaternary centres, subspecialisation has removed many secondary care consultants from more general circulation, and doctors have become more mobile in their careers, personal relationships between those in primary and secondary care have substantially diminished compared to those of days gone by.

In the confusing environment of repeated tendering processes, and of restructuring and reorganisation, it is also difficult for general practices to form reliable institutional relationships with secondary care providers.

This all contributes to make coordination between primary and secondary care more difficult. The Commonwealth Fund survey found that 79% of UK GPs reported that their patients had experienced problems in the past month because their care was not properly coordinated, which was significantly higher than the international average of 49%.[12]

The problem of coordinating care both with acute care providers and with community and social services is not unique to the United Kingdom, and improved integration of care is central to health policy in many developed nations; nevertheless, it is clearly an area that requires improvement in the United Kingdom.[12]

Not only is this poor coordination bad for the patient but also it increases the workload for GPs who must resolve the confusion that ensues. More fundamentally, it robs GPs of their ability to take ownership of their patients' care and derive the job satisfaction that comes from delivering and coordinating high-quality care.

CONCLUSION

There will always be pressure and stress in general practice as it is an intrinsic feature of caring for patients. However, the pressures are changing and whilst controlling some of these pressures, such as an aging population or rising patient expectation, is beyond the ability of any doctor or politician, controlling our response to these pressures is not.

In Chapters 1, 2 and 3, we have discussed many of the issues that contribute to GP burnout. The effect of these many different stressors on GPs has been likened to the effect of rising water temperature on a boiling frog.[16] The effect of the stressors can be insidious and, unless we are alert to them, action can be taken too late when the damage of burnout has already been done. There has been much research to discover what factors cause burnout amongst GPs; now we need ideas on how to tackle these problems so that we can either turn the heat down on the stove, or get out of the water altogether.

I WAS LUCKY FOR A NUMBER OF REASONS

Dr. Zoe Norris

GP Blogger and UK Chair of GPC Sessional Subcommittee

I was lucky for a number of reasons. Firstly, to have more experienced GP friends around me who had positive experiences of working for a medical chambers – a virtual practice set up with education, mentoring and peer support. They encouraged me to do this for a few months after I quit, and after the first meeting I realised I had laughed about work instead of crying, for the first time in months. That peer support made all the difference. But I was also disbelieving that I was the only person who was struggling like this. I couldn't believe I was an isolated case. I started speaking up and writing about the challenging environment I was working in, and suddenly was flooded with responses from other doctors and health care workers. The more I talked about it, the more support I got. It was a bizarre paradox and totally opposite to what I had expected. An exciting few months of blogging, media work, political campaigning followed.

Suddenly I had my dream job of teaching GP colleagues with an amazing team, brilliant support for my clinical work, the ability to try and support other GPs as an appraiser, and a national job in medical politics. It wasn't until further down the line that I started medication. I think the initial relief of moving quite quickly from a toxic environment, to one that I enjoyed with fewer demands emotionally meant I postponed getting the help I needed. I have used the term 'burnout' in the past, which implies my feelings and struggle was purely work related. To some extent that's true. But I recognise it has had lasting effects on me, and forced me to put a much higher value on my own self-care as a doctor. I deal with the inevitable guilt by telling myself that I am a much better doctor, and a better wife and mother for doing this. I also know the reality is that if I had made a mistake during that time, the lawyers and GMC wouldn't have cared how tired or over-worked I was. That's my one lasting message – you have to put yourself first sometimes. It feels impossible, but it's the only way to sustain your health.

REFERENCES

1. NHS England Analytical Service. *Improving general practice – A call to action. Evidence pack.* 2014.
2. Hobbs FR, Bankhead C, Mukhtar T, Stevens S, Perera-Salazar R, Holt T, Salisbury C, et al. Clinical workload in UK primary care: A retrospective analysis of 100 million consultations in England, 2007–14. *Lancet* 2016;387(10035):2323–30.

3. Gibson J, Checkland K, Coleman A, Hann M, Mccall R, Spooner S, Sutton M. *Eighth National GP Worklife Survey.* Policy Research Unit in Commissioning and the Healthcare System (PRUComm), London, 2015.
4. Dale J, Potter R, Owen K, Parsons N, Realpe A, Leach J. Retaining the general practitioner workforce in England: What matters to GPs? A cross-sectional study. *BMC Fam Pract* 2015;16:140.
5. Sansom A, Calitri R, Carter M, Campbell J. Understanding quit decisions in primary care: A qualitative study of older GPs. *BMJ Open* 2016;6(2):e010592.
6. The King's Fund. Future Trends in Time to Think Differently. 2012. The King's Fund: London. Accessed on 22 July, 2017.
7. Department of Health. *Report. Long-term conditions compendium of Information,* 3rd edn. Department of Health: London.
8. Royal College of General Practitioners. *Fair Funding for General Practice Campaign.* 2014. RCGP: London.
9. Bostock, N. GP partners' income fell a quarter in seven years from post-QOF peak. *GP Online.* 2014. Accessed on 22 July, 2017.
10. British Medical Association. Almost 300 GP practices facing closure and half of GP practices in England report GPs planning to desert the NHS, warns new BMA survey. *Press Release.* 2016. Accessed on 22 July, 2017.
11. Lind, S. More than 500 GP practices have closed in last five years, 'stark' Government figures reveal. *Pulse.* 2014. Accessed on 22 July, 2017.
12. Davies E, Martin S, Gershlick B. *Under pressure: What the Commonwealth Fund's 2015 International Survey of General Practitioners means for the UK.* 2016.
13. Omo, A. What's behind the rise in complaints about doctors from members of the public? *GMC Press Release.* 2014. Accessed on 22 July, 2017.
14. Leese B, Young R, Sibbald B. GP principals leaving practice in the UK. *Eur J Gen Pract* 2002;8:62–8.
15. Lateef F. Patient expectations and the paradigm shift of care in emergency medicine. *J Emerg Trauma Shock* 2011;4(2):163–7.
16. Doran N, Fox F, Rodham K, Taylor G, Harris M. Lost to the NHS: A mixed methods study of why GPs leave practice early in England. *Br J Gen Pract* 2016;66(643):e128–35.

4

Changing the system

DR. ADAM STATEN
The Red House Surgery, Bletchley, UK

The current era is unprecedented for the degree to which doctors have become politicised. The junior doctors' strikes of 2016 demonstrated a will amongst the medical profession to unite in action in a way which had not previously been seen and which startled the political classes.

Whilst the junior doctors may not have achieved all of their own aims, the action took the sting out of the intended contract negotiations for hospital consultants and for general practitioners (GPs), and stalled plans for yet another overhaul of working conditions in the National Health Service (NHS). The Department of Health had plans to change doctors' contracts throughout the NHS and decided to start with the group of doctors over whom it has the most power, and from whom it expected placid quiescence, but the industrial action largely derailed these plans.

It was momentous because doctors had finally united as a profession, with seniors overwhelmingly in support of the striking juniors, to demand a greater say over the running of the system in which they work.

However, whatever the strength of conviction of junior doctors, they were in a fundamentally weak position, dependent as they are on a monopoly employer to give them their training. Before completing their training, a junior doctor's alternatives to working in the NHS are really limited to two options, both more or less nuclear: emigrate or leave medicine. For many juniors these options are neither appealing nor practical.

Whilst it may not feel like it, GPs are in a far stronger position than their junior colleagues. Sitting in the consulting room of a general practice surgery it is easy to feel like a tiny, isolated cog in an enormous machine, but this is not so. GPs are the foundation upon which the entire structure of the NHS is built, and as a united entity, GPs have the power to topple the structure.

Independent contractor status makes GPs relatively free from the NHS, with the possibility, albeit daunting, of walking away from an NHS contract.

GPs already have many employment options including working for private or non-governmental providers, moving into different fields of medicine or leaving the country. But if GPs across the country worked in concert to leave the NHS, their options for continued employment in private health care would be almost limitless.

It often feels like we are subjects of the system, but this is not the case. The reality is that the system is subject to the will of general practice. Therefore, with resolve and unity, GPs can change the system in which they work.

CORPORATE POWER OF GPs

There are several professional bodies which can harness the collective power of GPs. At a local level the Local Medical Committee (LMC) represents the interests of GPs to the NHS authorities. They maintain connections with a wide range of other bodies including local health authorities, the NHS executive, and the British Medical Association (BMA), and they have a wide remit from ensuring equal opportunities to collaboration with the General Medical Council.

LMCs are well positioned to bring about change at both local and national levels, being small enough to remain responsive to the needs of those they represent locally but able to unite as a coalition to tackle national issues.

An example of what an LMC can achieve is the opt-out from the Quality Outcomes Framework (QOF) that the Somerset LMC negotiated in 2014. The QOF was replaced by a less rigid quality assurance scheme that could be better targeted to local, clinical needs and was less intrusive to normal practice. The move was subsequently replicated in other areas of the country and, on a larger scale, in Scotland where the link between the QOF and pay was scrapped after a vote at the Scottish LMC conference. Anecdotally, satisfaction levels amongst GPs who have adopted more nuanced quality assurance schemes are already on the rise.[1]

In 2016, the BMA launched its *Urgent Prescription for General Practice* campaign which urged the government to address many of the causes of stress and burnout in the profession. It risked being ignored, but the negotiation process was spurred on when the national LMC conference passed a motion to ballot members on industrial action, in the form of mass, undated resignation letters, if the measures outlined in the campaign were not accepted within 3 months.

NHS England subsequently agreed to discuss all of the proposals in the campaign which included measures to alleviate the cost of indemnity, increase the appointment lengths, limit GP workload, and provide financial support to struggling practices. This progress gives hope that there is now recognition of these problems and a governmental will to deal with them.

The LMCs provide a link between grassroots general practice and the BMA General Practitioners Committee (GPC) which is at the sharp end of negotiations between GPs and NHS England. This enables the GPC to bring about changes to the contract in response to the concerns of frontline GPs. Examples are the negotiated end of the deeply unpopular dementia direct enhanced service and the demise of the QOF.

The perceived failure of the negotiations in 1990, which resulted in contract imposition by then health secretary Kenneth Clarke, left many doctors feeling sceptical about the BMA's ability to bring about real change. But Kenneth Clarke himself described the doctors of the GPC as 'brilliant negotiators' and 'more difficult to deal with than the Rail Trade Unions' and the junior doctors' strike has recently demonstrated the BMA's ability to organise meaningful and powerful industrial action.[2]

In stark contrast to the junior doctors' strike, however, was the pension strike of 2012 which was poorly supported both by doctors and the general public. On the day of the strike, around three quarters of GP surgeries opened as normal. This lack of cohesion rendered the strikes absolutely ineffective and somewhat embarrassing. This demonstrates the need for GPs to engage in the political process as a collective if change is to be brought about.

Campaigns organised by the BMA and the GPC enable the Department of Health to be lobbied effectively, and there is no doubt that campaigns such as the *Urgent Prescription for General Practice* have brought the issues of a struggling workforce to the central attention of the powers that be.

As a membership body of professionals, rather than an industrial union, the Royal College of General Practitioners (RCGP) provides a softer touch approach to changing UK health care policy. Being both an academic and a professional institution, it can bring substantial weight to debates on health care policy and its policy team actively lobbies parliament on emerging issues that are problematic for GPs and for the patients that they care for.

Unlike the BMA and the LMCs, the RCGP can remain untainted by the grubby issue of contract negotiations and can remain upon the high horse of the duty of care, arguing that what is good for general practice is good for NHS patients. The campaign *Put Patients First: Back General Practice* was the first political campaign in the RCGP's history. It sought to improve funding to general practice, and the campaign was influential in shaping NHS England's *GP Forward View* which proposed increasing the funding to general practice to more than 10% of the total NHS budget.

Working separately or in concert, these three bodies provide powerful outlets for GPs to voice their concerns and to influence change in the entire NHS system, but they rely on the continued and enthusiastic engagement of their members to inform and bring about this change.

VALUE OF THE CCGs

When Clinical Commissioning Groups were created following the Health and Social Care Act of 2012, the grey beards of general practice rolled their collective eyes. Many of those who had experienced the rise and fall of fundholding, total purchasing, practice-based commissioning, and the primary care groups and trusts had little enthusiasm for the latest incarnation of the NHS internal market.

The primary care trusts had seen an all-time low in clinical engagement, and there was a real danger that GPs would not engage fully with the CCGs.[3] To some, CCGs are a particularly hard sell as they bring with them an extra burden of work that many fear will itself contribute to GP burnout, but with two thirds of the NHS budget placed in the hands of the new CCGs there can be little doubt that they offer a definite opportunity for GPs to influence the system in which they work.[4]

The development of CCGs is the first time that GPs have been placed truly at the forefront of commissioning, and they afford commissioners more autonomy to shape local services than previous forms of commissioning.[5,6]

Evidence suggests that CCGs have managed to secure more engagement than previous forms of commissioning,[7] and this is crucial because commissioning is only effective if GPs engage with it.[7] Research conducted by the King's Fund has found that more than 70% of GPs feel engaged with the CCGs, with the majority of GPs seeing the CCGs as an influential part of the local health economy. And, as the CCGs have developed, GP leaders working within them have grown more confident in making important decisions to change the way that primary care is organised in their local area.[5]

There are, however, many sceptics, and it was notable in the research that the feeling of engagement was significantly lower amongst GPs with no formal role in the CCG. Many of those without a role still feel that it is difficult to influence decisions made by their CCG. This risks division between those within the CCG structure and those without. Such division could create a group of GPs who feel disenfranchised and another group, working within the CCG, who are no longer responsive to the needs of their colleagues and who are in danger of going native with the political super structure. Therefore, those GPs who feel disengaged must be reached out to.

Running the CCGs without doubt burdens GPs with a great deal of extra work, but it is possible to make this system work for GPs, improve life at work and thereby reduce overall occupational stress. To achieve this, services should be commissioned that are targeted at those areas of primary care that contribute most to workplace stress. In this respect the needs of GPs and the needs of patients frequently overlap as it is those most in need, whether that need is medical, social or emotional, who are the source of the greatest amount of GP workload.

With 211 CCGs across the country, all independently commissioning services, there are already a large number of projects underway which may serve to reduce the pressure from some of the key stressors contributing to burnout.

For example, poor coordination of care is a key factor in creating stress, and the Sutton CCG responded to complex care pathways and poorly coordinated mental health services by commissioning a single referral point through which all patients with mental health needs, whether that be for bereavement counselling or same day psychiatric assessment, could be triaged.

Numerous CCGs have commissioned services to help deal with the issues surrounding multi-morbid, elderly patients. In Greenwich 'care navigators' direct people with complex conditions to local services without the need to visit their GP or hospital.[4]

Social prescribing is being explored by many CCGs, such as in Gloucestershire, as a means of reducing the burden of patients attending their GP with non-medical issues and thereby reducing the dependence of the local population on their family doctors.

It is probably too early to say whether these schemes will be truly effective in reducing the workload of GPs, but with the enormous scope for experimentation and the sharing of knowledge between CCGs it seems likely that some helpful services will be developed which will not only offset the workload of running the CCG but also improve the working life of GPs.

Although the CCG model may not have been one that many GPs would have chosen, it is the model with which we must currently work. That being so, it will be best for doctors and patients alike if GPs fully engage and take the opportunity that CCGs provide to bring about real change in the system.

GP FEDERATIONS

GP federations were first proposed in the RCGP's *Roadmap* for general practice in 2007. They were seen as a way for GPs to counter the challenges of the NHS internal market and to enable GPs to guide the development of services that would be best suited to their local community.[8]

The idea was expanded in the RCGP's publication *Primary Care Federations: Putting Patients First* in 2008 in which it was argued that the federation of practices would make general practice more financially viable and sustainable for the future by enabling GPs to compete with larger organisations in tendering for services. Federations would enable GPs to offer a wider range of diagnostics and treatments in a cost-effective way, as well as allowing patients to receive more advanced levels of care in the familiar environment of local general practices. Economies of scale could be introduced, particularly with regard to backroom functions, which would enable GPs to bring more services out of the hospital and into the community, bringing new streams of income into surgeries and so alleviating the financial pressures that cause so much stress and difficulty within general practice.

BENEFITS OF GP FEDERATIONS

- Introducing cost efficiency and economies of scale
- Improving service integration across practices and other providers
- Enabling practices to tender for new services
- Developing training and education capacity
- Allowing GPs to diversify and pool their skills
- Improving quality and reducing health inequalities

At an individual level, federations would encourage GPs to diversify their skill set, developing specialist interests, so that practices could pool the abilities of their constituent doctors to offer this greater range of services.[9] The federations would therefore offer a wide range of benefits, from improving the financial viability of practices to allowing GPs to re-invigorate their careers by developing special interests.

The idea of forming federations is not unique to the United Kingdom, and organisations similar to federations have existed in other countries for some time. In New Zealand, practices have formed themselves into Independent Practice Associations since the early 1990s, and this has enabled GPs to direct resources more effectively to instigate disease management programmes, improve immunisation rates and make savings in costs such as laboratory fees.[10] Practices have also grouped together to achieve similar goals in countries such as Spain, Portugal, Italy and Australia.[11]

In 2010, the RCGP commissioned a toolkit to assist practices with the process of federating, and in subsequent years GP practices have increasingly sought to collaborate with one another across the country.[12]

By creating economies of scale, federations allow GPs to tender for services in a way that would simply not be possible at an individual practice level. This allows GPs to combat the erosion of income caused when private companies undercut the tenders of individual practices to cherry pick services such as vaccinations, services that are easy to deliver and highly profitable, leaving GPs to deliver more complex, less profitable, but no less essential services.

Not only do federations allow GPs to prevent the erosion of their traditional streams of income, but they have also enabled GPs to derive income by delivering services that are normally delivered in the hospital. For example, the Milton Keynes GP federation now delivers services such as pre-op assessment, fast track treatments of deep vein thromboses and injectable pain management which had previously been the preserve of the local hospital.

GP federations have also allowed groups of practices to commit funds toward tackling the workforce issues that are proving so problematic nationwide. For example, the Suffolk GP federation has invested in developing plans to provide pre-retirement support for GPs to retain them within the workforce. They are also planning to create a locum chambers with the specific intention of capturing the capabilities of recently retired GPs who wish to continue working but with a reduced workload and no management responsibilities.

The creation of federations, in conjunction with the creation of the CCGs, places GPs on both sides of the purchaser–provider split and in an incredibly strong position to influence local service provision in a way that could be both financially profitable and personally satisfying. Done well, this could go a long way to combating stress amongst GPs.

HARNESSING SOCIAL MEDIA

As discussed in Chapter 2, the negative media portrayal of GPs, and the wider medical profession, has been identified as a source of real stress amongst GPs and a contributory factor in the decision of many GPs to leave general practice.[13] The motivation for such critical coverage is not always obvious but includes the political agenda of particular publications, perceived government pressure on state-funded outlets such as the British Broadcasting Corporation, and the modern pressures of journalism when publicity is easier to attract with bad news than with good news. Often the motivation seems to be simple spite.

As former chancellor Nigel Lawson said, the NHS 'is the nearest thing the English have to a religion' and so stories about health always get plenty of coverage in the United Kingdom. This relentless criticism from the mainstream media can be incredibly demoralising and gives the perception that the general public is at odds with the medical profession, thus undermining the traditional values of the patient–doctor relationship which is reliant on trust and respect in both directions. Whilst penetrating mainstream media platforms to express a more balanced opinion can be very difficult for the average GP, we are fortunate now to have an alternative means of expressing ourselves in the form of social media.

The junior doctors' strike again provides a good example of this in action. *The Sun* newspaper ran a campaign during the strikes to undermine the junior doctors, the notorious 'Moet Medics' campaign which sought to portray junior doctors as cosseted sybarites. This was effectively undone by the social media response of junior doctors. Whilst many newspapers and TV programmes sought to portray the strikes in a negative light, the noise on social media made it evident that there was in reality overwhelming public support for the protest, and this reinforced the resolve of the juniors and helped to legitimise the strikes.

The beauty of social media, whether that is writing blogs, sending tweets or posting on social media sites, is that it opens up a two-way dialogue allowing doctors to converse with the public and put across nuanced and detailed arguments.

Because well-written and interesting articles can be so widely shared, it is possible for writers to reach an enormous audience within a matter of minutes even if the initial platform on which an article is written is relatively obscure.

Not only can there be an incredible amount of personal catharsis in expressing thoughts and concerns in this way, but it is also a genuinely effective means of getting important messages about the state of general practice out to the public. There is also potential for this to create a virtuous circle of media coverage as the mainstream media derives much of its content from what is trending on social media.

This can be done at a smaller and more local scale as well. With many patients now accessing appointments online, the practice website is now an ideal platform for local GPs to write blogs in which they can educate their patients and keep them informed about local health issues. Providing education from a trusted source at the point of booking an appointment may be a powerful tool in obviating the need for some of those appointments.

Social media presents doctors with an opportunity to educate patients and influence public opinion which will ultimately dictate the direction in which services are taken.

CONCLUSION

It is not easy to change a system as large as the NHS, but it is not impossible. The mechanisms by which change can be achieved, such as the GPC, the CCGs and the federations, already exist, and one could argue that the system has been tipped in the favour of GPs who are now in the powerful position of straddling the purchaser–provider split. Thus, it is possible that some truly revolutionary ways of working and delivering care could be developed. Furthermore, these new models of working can be tailored specifically to the local population and to those issues that create most stress for GPs.

The key to driving this change is engagement. The system will not change by itself and nor will it be changed to the advantage of general practice if GPs remain on the outside slinging mud or, worse, suffering silently. By engaging with bodies such as the LMCs, the BMA and the RCGP, and by publicising these issues to a public who may not be aware that they exist, health care policy can be changed.

The system needs GPs, but it will not have them much longer if things carry on as they are. The issues that put general practice under so much pressure must be dealt with in one way or another if the NHS is to survive and we, as GPs, can either wait until the system is so damaged that dealing with the issues is unavoidable or we can engage, unite and mobilise to improve things before they get worse.

REFERENCES

1. Twaddell, I. What is life like post QOF? Pulse. 2016. http://www.pulseto-day.co.uk/your-practice/qof/what-is-life-like-postqof/20032555.article. Accessed on 22 July, 2017.
2. BMA. *Continuity in a changing world: 100 years of GP representative bodies.* British Medical Association: London. 2012.
3. Perkins N, Coleman A, Wright M, Gadsby E, McDermott I, Petsoulas C, Checkland K. The 'added value' GPs bring to commissioning: A qualitative study in primary care. *Br J Gen Pract* 2014;64(628):e728–34. doi:10.3399/bjgp14X682321.
4. NHS Clinical Commisioners. About CCGs. http://www.nhscc.org/ccgs/. Accessed on 22 July, 2017.
5. The King's Fund. *Has clinical commissioning found its voice? GP perspectives on their CCGs.* The King's Fund: London. 2016.
6. Checkland K, Coleman A, McDermott I, Segar J, Miller R, Petsoulas C, Wallace A, Harrison S, Peckham S. Primary care-led commissioning: Applying lessons from the past to the early development of clinical commissioning groups in England. *Br J Gen Pract.* 2013;63(614):e611–19. doi:10.3399/bjgp13X671597.
7. The King's Fund. *Clinical commissioning: GPs in charge.* The Kings Fund: London. 2016.

8. RCGP. *The future direction: Roadmap.* Royal College of General Practitioners: London. 2007. http://www.rcgp.org.uk/policy/rcgp-policy-areas/~/media/Files/Policy/A-Z-policy/the_future_direction_rcgp_roadmap.ashx. Accessed on 22 July, 2017.

9. RCGP. *Primary care federations: Putting patients first.* Royal College of General Practitioners: London. 2008.

10. Malcolm L. New Zealand's independent practitioner associations: A working model of clinical governance in primary care? *BMJ* 1999;319:1340–2.

11. Roland M. *The Future of Primary Care – Keynote speech*, WONCA. 2016. http://www.woncaeurope2016.com/images/Keynote-powerpoints/Martin-Roland-Keynote-Hall-A-Friday-09.pdf. Accessed on 22 July, 2017.

12. The King's Fund. *Primary care federations toolkit.* The King's Fund: London. 2010.

13. Doran N, Fox F, Rodham K, Taylor G, Harris M. Lost to the NHS: A mixed methods study of why GPs leave practice early in England. *Br J Gen Pract.* 2016;66(643):e128–35.

5

Changing the way we work

DR. ADAM STATEN
The Red House Surgery, Bletchley, UK

Whatever changes may lie in store for the structure and organisation of general practice, the shifting demographics of the UK population make it inevitable that general practitioners (GPs) will have to adapt to new pressures. Rising expectations, increasingly complex patients and a growing population will always challenge us.

It will not simply be enough to change the system in which we work; we must also change the way we work within it. Efficiencies in time, money and psychological burden can be made by approaching the old issues of primary care in fresh ways.

The small business model of general practice, the larger units of GP federations and the overarching unity of the specialty make general practice fertile grounds for innovation at a small, medium and large scale, and there is scope for minor tweaks to what we already do and for blue sky thinking to create completely new models of care.

EMBRACING TECHNOLOGY

The use of technology in one form or another is ubiquitous within UK general practice, but with regard to our use of technology, we need to ask two questions: (1) Are we using the best available technologies to solve our problems? and (2) Are we using our technology in the best way?

Interacting with the practice computer system

A simple example of a piece of technology which is frequently very badly used is the computer keyboard. With 98% of GPs in the United Kingdom using electronic medical records, almost all our patient interactions result in typing (Figure 5.1).[1] Yet how many GPs touch type proficiently? A GP who types by the 'hunt and peck'

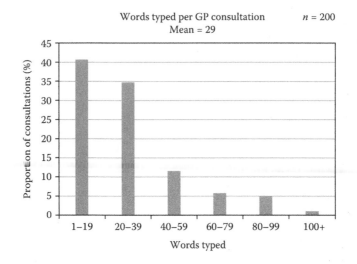

Figure 5.1 Words Typed per GP Consultation. (From www.england.nhs.uk/wp-content/uploads/2016/03/releas-capcty-6-topic-sht-6-3.pdf)

method can type about 30 words per minute. An audit of 200 consultations found that a GP who types likes this could save about 17 min a day by learning how to touch type proficiently, assuming a consultation rate of 40 patients each day.[2] Touch typing is a skill that can be learned over 2–4 weeks with a few minutes of effort each day, and it is a skill that can save time in every consultation and allow doctors to write more thorough, litigation proof notes, and yet few of us take the time to learn it.

The use of electronic medical records (EMRs) in the United Kingdom is amongst the highest in the world.[1] EMRs allow the workload of general practice to be stream-lined in several ways such as improved data analysis, ease of access to test results and correspondence, electronic prescribing and the sharing of patient records across community services to improve coordination of care. However, there is marked vari-ability in the exploitation of these capabilities across the country; for example, 78% of practices in London can transfer prescriptions electronically to the pharmacy com-pared to just 3% in Northern Ireland, and only 31% of practices in Wales order lab tests electronically compared to 91% in England (outside of London).[1]

Often, an EMR system is not used to the best of its capabilities. For example many GPs take printed summaries of patient notes to home visits, requiring them to type notes up when they get back to the surgery, but EMR systems, such as EMIS, are often capable of being used remotely on laptops, tablets and smart-phones. Remote access can also allow GPs to go through pathology results and correspondence from home, perhaps after having arrived home in time to put the children to bed or have dinner with the family.

Similarly, voice recognition technology can be used to dictate directly into patient notes, obviating the need to type at all and enabling GPs to make notes at a much greater speed than even a proficient touch typist.

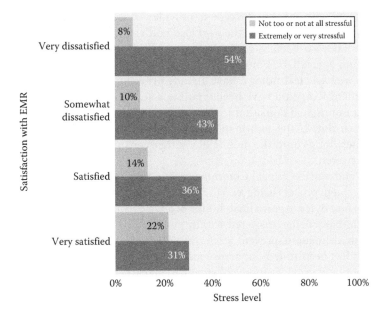

Figure 5.2 Relationship between GPs' Satisfaction with Their EMR and How Stressful They Find Their Job. (From Davies, E. et al., *Under Pressure: What the Commonwealth Fund's 2015 International Survey of General Practitioners Means for the UK*, http://www.health.org.uk/publication/under-pressure#sthash.3qqLghqH.dpuf, 2016.)

Muddling through with EMR technology with which you are familiar, but which may not be the best available, is not just a matter of streamlining minor processes in the working day. There is a clear correlation between levels of satisfaction with EMR systems and with perceived levels of occupational stress (see Figure 5.2).[1] The capital investment in new EMR technology is therefore almost certainly justified from the perspective of preventing burnout.

Communicating via new technologies

Today, patients have many more means by which they can contact us than in the past, yet most surgeries are still limited to either face-to-face consultations or telephone consultations. In particular, the younger cohort of our patients are familiar and comfortable with communication via video phone, text or email, and a study examining the use of these technologies to provide virtual clinics for young diabetic patients found that their use reduced non-attendance rates from 30%–50% to 16% compared to usual care.[3]

Skype™, a free Internet-based videophone application, has been well researched for use in several areas including providing remote health care to refugees and providing psychotherapy, and it has even been effective when used for orthopaedic follow-up.[4–6] General practices in the United Kingdom have also experimented with the use of Skype to provide virtual ward rounds at nursing homes in an attempt to reduce the workload burden of nursing homes.

Skype has also been suggested as a means by which GPs could access advice from specialists, but other means of accessing specialist advice, reliant on more basic technology, have already proven very effective. Fifty areas in the United Kingdom have been trialling a scheme by which each specialism has a nominated consultant who can be contacted for immediate phone advice each day. If the nominated consultant is unable to answer, the call immediately loops onto the mobile of another consultant and so on until the call is answered.

The Wandsworth Clinical Commissioning Group (CCG) has trialled a referral management process using a secure email system by which consultants can be contacted for advice. Approximately 60% of advice requests are answered within 24 h, with many being answered within minutes or hours, and approximately 58% of advice requests prevent a referral.[7] The scheme has proved so successful that it has been rolled out across many CCGs in South West London. The scheme not only provides more coherent patient care, and reduces referrals, but also enhances the relationships between GPs and specialists and contributes to education and professional development. This also allows GPs to retain ownership and control of their patient's care which contributes to continuity of care and to job satisfaction.

Telehealth

A more contentious area in which technology has been trialled is telehealth. Telehealth is the use of monitoring technology in the patient's home to provide biometric data, in conditions such as chronic obstructive pulmonary disease, diabetes or hypertension, which can be remotely relayed to a health care professional to monitor the patient's status and intervene if necessary. GPs have often been sceptical about such schemes, feeling that it will probably add to workload rather than ease it, but further research has suggested that, whilst telehealth schemes do not reduce patient contact with GPs, they do not actually add to GP workload.[8,9]

A large scale trial, the Whole Systems Demonstrator programme, found that telehealth, in the form trialled, was not cost effective compared to routine care, but a major weakness of this, and other telehealth studies, is that the biometric data are usually not sent to the GP.[10] This is something that clearly warrants some research before the potential impact of telehealth on general practice can be assessed.

We are unlikely to have heard the final word on telehealth, particularly as technologies change, evolve and become cheaper, and it seems probable that technology will have some role to play in empowering patients to manage their own conditions and reducing the need to contact their GPs.

Technology can help us practice more flexibly, allowing us to adapt to new challenges and manage our workload more effectively. New applications for technology should be actively sought and trialled by GPs to help overcome the many obstacles and difficulties we face in daily practice.

INCREASING THE SKILL MIX IN PRIMARY CARE

The delivery of primary care is increasing in complexity, and any attempt by GPs to deliver primary care in isolation is doomed to failure. There are many primary care tasks that do not need the skills or training of a GP, and there are many tasks that are carried out better by other health professionals.[11] If we are to offer a wider range of services in a coherent way then we need to increase the skill mix of our primary care teams. This idea was central to the recommendations of the primary care workforce commission report, *The Future of Primary Care: Building Teams for Tomorrow.*[12]

By some estimates the GP workload could be cut by up to 20% by more effective use of other health professionals, so it is well worth considering bringing an increasing variety of skills into our surgeries.[13] The range of professionals working in general practice internationally can be quite different to that commonly found in UK practices and, in some countries, it is common for social workers, psychiatric nurses, physiotherapists, dentists and pharmacists to work alongside GPs.[14]

Physiotherapists

In 2015 the Chartered Society of Physiotherapists made a positive bid to be more involved in primary care. With up to 3 of every 10 GP appointments used for musculoskeletal issues, they estimated that around 100 million GP appointments could be freed up each year if physiotherapists were made the first point of contact for musculoskeletal problems. What's more, the service would be delivered more cost effectively.[15]

Such a shift in workload would rely on allowing patients to self-refer to physiotherapy and England, where only 31% of CCGs have any self-referral for physiotherapy, lags significantly behind Scotland where 86% of areas allow full self-referral, and the remaining areas have partial self-referral schemes.[15]

The Royal College of General Practitioners was sceptical about the commissioning of such services, citing evidence that a pilot scheme in the Midlands had been utterly swamped by demand, but there is evidence that, when services are refined by telephone triage, direct access physiotherapy is effective and cost effective.[16,17] A scheme in Torbay allowing self-referral cut waiting times for physiotherapy from 10 weeks to less than 3 days for 90% of patients.[15]

Pharmacist and medicines management

The use of pharmacists, particularly for face-to-face consultations, within general practice surgeries remains relatively unusual in the United Kingdom. There are however practices that have been using pharmacists, in some cases as partners in the practice, for many years with great effect. An example of this arrangement is the Wallingbrook Health Group in Devon which has had a clinical pharmacist partner since 2004. Here the pharmacist helps patients to manage their own conditions, optimises medications, helps manage patients with long-term, stable conditions and informs practice medication policies. The practice estimates that the pharmacist has been instrumental in reducing demand for GP appointments by up to 20–30%.[18]

Based on cases such as the Wallingbrook Health Group, the closer inclusion of clinical pharmacists in primary care teams was also a key recommendation in *The Future of Primary Care: Creating Teams for Tomorrow*. It was envisaged that pharmacists, particularly those with a prescribing role, should be used to help with medication reviews, optimisation of medications and repeat prescriptions; review of post hospital discharge; and management of complex care home residents. To this end, National Health Service (NHS) England has funded a pilot of 403 new clinical pharmacist posts across 73 sites.[19]

The cost of medication errors in both human and financial terms is not inconsiderable. Up to 5% of general practice prescriptions contain errors and 0.18% of these are potentially serious.[20] The cost to the NHS of hospital admissions directly resulting from adverse drug reactions is thought to be £440 million each year and between 2005 and 2010, 822 medication errors resulted in death or severe harm.[20] With rising polypharmacy, it is not hard to see how the close inclusion of a clinical pharmacist in the primary care team could reduce workload and stress.

Physician associates

A category of professional that will be less familiar to many working in general practice than physios and pharmacists is the physician associate (PA). Formerly known as a physician assistant, this new breed of allied health professional are people who possess a science degree and have then undergone an intensive 2-year training course in the medical model. They have been established in the United States for around 40 years and there are around 80,000 working in the United States at present.[21] However, here in the United Kingdom, there are currently only a few hundred, but seen as a partial solution to the work force crisis, the funding tap has been turned on and we are likely to see many more in the coming years.[21]

Their introduction into general practice is not without controversy, with many arguing that the government is using them as a budget means of plugging workforce gaps. With such limited numbers currently working in general practice, there are few robust studies assessing how well PAs work within UK primary care, but one study concluded that the processes and outcomes of PA and GP appointments were the same, with a cost saving from the PA appointments.[22] The endpoint in this study was repeat attendance within 14 days, and the study authors conceded that the PAs were seeing younger and less complex patients and had appointment lengths of 15 or 20 min rather than 10 min.

For many this study will not establish the value of PAs within the primary care workforce, but to dismiss these intelligent and educated people out of hand is probably a mistake. Crucially, PAs are trained to be *dependent* practitioners. Some see this as a disadvantage, presenting a risk of burdening their supervising GP with more work, but it also means that their role can be determined by those doctors on whom they are dependent and therefore tailored to the needs of that doctor.

Perhaps PAs will find their primary care niche working in a 'medical assistant' role. Medical assistants are another type of US health care professional who work doing basic procedures, assisting in the coordination of chronic disease management and reviewing test results and correspondence, flagging those of importance for review by the doctor. In a paper boldly titled, *In Search of Joy in Practice*, medical assistants were identified as a means of doctors liberating themselves from administration, and its associated stress, and focusing more on direct patient care.[23]

Mental health workers

The burden of mental health problems is large in primary care, and it has long been argued that mental health professionals, usually in the form of psychiatric nurses, should be more integral to the primary care team. Back in 1997 the Maudsley Hospital published a discussion paper recommending that psychiatric nurses be relieved of their supportive role to free them up to provide active treatments, such as cognitive behavioural therapy, within primary care teams.[24] In the two decades since, this vision has largely not been realised but in many countries, such as the Netherlands, it is far more common for mental health nurses to work in GP surgeries.

A large Dutch study examining the impact of mental health nurses in primary care did not find that the nurses particularly ease the workload of GPs, or cause patients suffering with mental health problems to consult with their GPs less, but it did find that the nurses offered the benefit of long extra appointments that could be used therapeutically.[25] Perhaps this suggests that it is not necessary for mental health nurses to be located within GP surgeries; rather, they may be best left under the umbrella of organisations such as Improving Access to Psychological Therapies, but it does identify the therapeutic value of mental health nurses within the primary care setup.

The model of GPs working alongside practice nurses and nurse practitioners can only be stretched so far and can only offer so many services. The world of health care is full of skilled and highly trained people and, as yet, we are probably not making best use of our resources. To relieve ourselves of the stresses of an increasingly complex world, it is essential that we learn to find a way of using our resources more effectively.

INNOVATIVE MODELS OF SEEING PATIENTS

The patient has a problem, the patient books an appointment to see their GP, the GP sees the patient in the consultation room. So it was, so it is, but so shall it always be? The traditional model of seeing patients in general practice was developed in an era of GPs working in relative solitude with no effective alternative means of communicating with their patients. With an expanded team, and with new technology at our disposal, it stands to reason that the way in which we see patients should also evolve.

There is probably no one-size-fits-all solution to managing workload, but there is already a great deal of experimentation going on around the country, the results of which, if shared, should allow practices to take a pick-and-mix approach to providing an effective service for their patients. Practices should be willing to test and adjust to their own circumstances, seeking novel solutions to individual pressures, and developing their own ways of seeing their patients.

Telephone triage

Perhaps the most common change in practice of the past two decades is the use of telephone triage by many surgeries. Telephone triage of those patients requesting same-day appointments has been embraced by many GPs, but the evidence supporting it is somewhat equivocal. There is good evidence showing that patients find telephone consultations an acceptable alternative to face-to-face appointments and that telephone appointments save time on the index day of a request for an appointment, but there is also evidence that this time saving is offset by higher rates of re-consultation in the period after triage.[26-29]

The ESTEEM trial[29] is the most recent and the largest trial looking at the benefits or otherwise of telephone triage. Its authors concluded that, overall number of primary care contacts in the 28 days following the initial request for an appointment was increased if the triage was conducted by a GP, and was further increased if the triage was nurse led. There was also no cost savings with telephone triage. These results surprised and dismayed many who advocate telephone triage who report resolving 60% of problems over the phone, and reducing overall workload by up to 35%, with an increase in patient continuity, and a sense of greater control for the doctors which is clearly very important in maintaining job satisfaction and avoiding burnout.[30]

The ESTEEM trial has faced criticism for testing one component of the telephone triage system, rather than measuring systemic effects, and further large-scale trials are planned to tease out what the benefits of telephone triage truly are.[30]

However, one possible problem with telephone triage is that patients are still being triaged into a traditional system with limited options available to the triaging doctor. Triage could be even more effective if the GP had a greater repertoire of services at his or her disposal. The primary care workforce commission report envisaged GPs working in a more consultative role, overseeing a surrounding team of allied health professionals as outlined in the previous section.[31]

The Roundhouse Model

The idea of a GP operating in a triaging, overseeing and trouble-shooting capacity has been taken to its extreme in a proposed new model of general practice known as the 'Roundhouse Model' (see Figure 5.3). This model sees GPs operating both physically and organisationally at the centre of an allied team of professionals

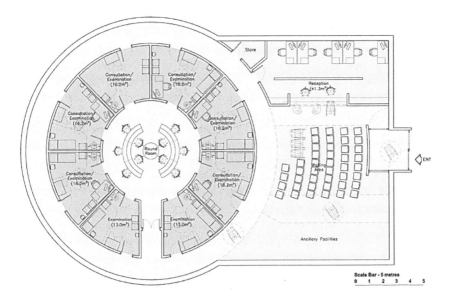

Figure 5.3 The 'Roundhouse'. (From Lewis, D.M. et al., *Br. J. Gen. Pract.*, 66, 646, 2016. With permission.)

in a purpose built building with psychiatric nurses, orthopaedic practitioners, nurses and nurse practitioners, pharmacists and physicians associates.[32] Sitting in the 'roundroom' is the 'consultant primary care physician', helping nurses perform telephone triage, performing email consultations and overseeing the roundhouse. No doubt this is a role that some GPs would relish but many might miss the routine, direct contact with their patients and, obviously, adopting this model in this exact format would bring with it some eye-watering set-up costs.

Shared medical appointments

A less revolutionary new means of seeing patients, and one that is growing both in its popularity and evidence base, is the 'shared medical appointment'. In essence these are group educational sessions, typically lasting around 90 min, that are used to improve patient wellbeing and empower patients to manage their own conditions. So, rather than teach individual patients the same lessons about their illnesses over and over again throughout the day, overall clinician time is saved by giving much more detailed education to a group of patients. This gives the added benefit of coincidentally providing a peer support network for patients.

Shared medical appointments have been used, and found to be effective, in a wide range of conditions such as diabetes, asthma, pregnancy, and liver disease. Evidence suggests that patients are more satisfied with care delivered via shared appointments compared to usual care, and outcomes are good in terms of health and the patient's ability to self-manage.[33,34] Not only are there benefits in time saved for the doctor, but also doctors report finding the experience professionally satisfying.[35]

The virtual ward and coordination of care

The challenge of managing medically complex patients is one that may also be amenable to new ways of working. The concept of the 'virtual ward' remains slightly amorphous in the literature. In one incarnation of the idea that was trialled by the Devon and Torbay PCT (now CCG) for several years from 2010, the virtual ward consisted of care for patients at high risk of admission being coordinated by a 'care co-ordinator' and a monthly multidisciplinary team meeting being held to organise that care and review progress. The idea built on good relationships between general practice, community services and the voluntary sector and aimed to provide holistic and personalised care plans whilst cutting out the duplication of effort that can occur with poorly coordinated care.[36]

Early data from the trial suggested reduced rates of emergency admission and fewer requirements for nursing home placements, but later data were more equivocal. Unfortunately, the project was severely hampered by changes in clinical governance procedures and organisational structure. Ultimately, the Nuffield Trust who analysed the scheme concluded that they were unable to say whether virtual wards worked, but new ideas such as this, which help with making the coordination of multiple services more efficient and more coherent, will certainly be needed in the coming years.[37]

Co-ordination of care is not only a problem between services; providing continuous care for patients within a practice can sometimes pose a challenge, particularly with the increasing move to part-time work and portfolio careers amongst GPs. This lack of continuity can be frustrating for doctors and patients alike with fragmented care, duplication of effort and the loss of the satisfaction of seeing problems through to their conclusion. Even the uncertainty of whether an unwell patient is being followed up properly can be stressful for the absent, part-time doctor.

To combat this stress, a new practice of forming 'micro teams' is emerging.[38] Within a surgery doctors and nurses form smaller sub-teams. If a patient is unable to book with their usual or preferred GP then they are given an appointment with another member of the micro team. Whilst this does not guarantee continuity with a particular doctor, it does give continuity with a small group of doctors who can become familiar with one another's ways of practicing and provide better, continuous care which gives piece of mind to both the doctor and the patient.

CONCLUSION

It is easy to become buried beneath a heavy workload and working hard can make it difficult to think about working differently. The ways in which we work, the teams in which we work and even the technologies with which we work are familiar, but they are not immutable. On the surface, familiarity brings comfort, but the evidence suggests that the familiar is breaking general practice and breaking GPs.

To change working practices is a daunting move and to hire new team members and update technology at times of financial difficulty is a brave move, but to avoid the risk of burnout these are moves that are becoming more or less essential.

REFERENCES

1. Davies E, Martin S, Gershlick B. *Under pressure: What the Commonwealth Fund's 2015 International Survey of General Practitioners means for the UK.* 2016. http://www.health.org.uk/sites/health/files/UnderPressure.pdf. Accessed on 23 July, 2017.

2. NHS England. Releasing Capacity in General Practice (10 High Impact Actions), 6.3 Topic Sheet 3 – Touch Typing and Speed Reading. NHS England: Leeds. 2016. https://www.england.nhs.uk/wp-content/uploads/2016/03/releas-capcty-6-topic-sht-6-3.pdf. Accessed on 23 July, 2017.

3. Mayor, S. Use texts, apps, and Skype to keep young people with diabetes engaged with services, says guidance. *BMJ.* 2016;352:i394.

4. Schulz TR, Richards M, Gasko H, Lohrey J, Hibbert ME, Biggs BA. Telehealth: Experience of the first 120 consultations delivered from a new refugee telehealth clinic. *Intern Med J.* 2014;44(10):981–5.

5. Edirippulige S, Levandovskaya M, Prishutova A. A qualitative study of the use of Skype for psychotherapy consultations in the Ukraine. *J Telemed Telecare* 2013;19(7):376–8.

6. Good DW, Lui DF, Leonard M, Morris S, McElwain JP. Skype: A tool for functional assessment in orthopaedic research. *J Telemed Telecare* 2012;18(2):94–8.

7. Wandsworth CCG. Wandsworth CCG: Reducing Outpatient Referrals. http://www.kinesisgp.co.uk/Content/_KINESISGP/Uploads/Wandsworth_CCG_Case%20Study.pdf. Accessed on 23 July, 2017.

8. MacNeill V, Sanders C, Fitzpatrick R, Hendy J, Barlow J, Knapp M, Rogers A, Bardsley M, Newman SP. Experiences of front-line health professionals in the delivery of telehealth: A qualitative study. *Br J Gen Pract* 2014;64(624):e401–7. doi: 10.3399/bjgp14X680485.

9. Bardsley M, Steventon A, Doll H. Impact of telehealth on general practice contacts: Findings from the whole systems demonstrator cluster randomised trial. *BMC Health Serv Res* 2013;13:395.

10. Henderson C, Knapp M, Fernández JL, Beecham J, Hirani SP, Cartwright M, Rixon L, et al. Cost effectiveness of telehealth for patients with long term conditions (Whole Systems Demonstrator telehealth questionnaire study): Nested economic evaluation in a pragmatic, cluster randomised controlled trial. *BMJ* 2013;346:f1035.

11. Roland M. *The future of primary care – Keynote speech.* WONCA. 2016. http://www.woncaeurope2016.com/images/Keynote-powerpoints/Martin-Roland-Keynote-Hall-A-Friday-09.pdf. Accessed on 23 July, 2017.

12. Health Education England. *The future of primary care: Creating teams for tomorrow.* http://hee.nhs.uk/wp-content/blogs.dir/321/files/2015/07/The-future-of-primary-care.pdf. Accessed on 23 July, 2017.

13. Chan, S. Exclusive: Pharmacists and physiotherapists 'could reduce GP workload by 20%'. *GP Online*. 2015. http://www.gponline.com/exclusive-pharmacists-physiotherapists-couldreduce-gp-workload-20/article/1348950. Accessed on 23 July, 2017.

14. Groenewegen P, Heinemann S, Greß S, Schäfer W. Primary care practice composition in 34 countries. *Health Policy* 2015;119(12):1576–83.

15. Chartered Society of Physiotherapists. Place physiotherapists on the frontline to free up millions of GP appointments, says CSP. *Press Release*. 2015. http://www.csp.org.uk/press-releases/2015/04/22/place-physio-therapistsfrontline-free-millions-gp-appointments-says-csp. Accessed on 23 July, 2017.

16. Griffiths, E. Physiotherapists' call for patient self-referral shot down by RCGP. *Pulse*. 2015. http://www.pulsetoday.co.uk/news/clinical-news/phys-iotherapists-callfor-patient-self-referral-shot-down-by-rcgp/20009792.fullarticle. Accessed on 23 July, 2017.

17. Mallett R, Bakker E, Burton M. Is physiotherapy self-referral with tele-phone triage viable, cost-effective and beneficial to Musculoskeletal outpatients in a primary care setting? *Musculoskeletal Care* 2014;12(4):251–60.

18. NHS England. Case study: Clinical pharmacists in general practice. 2015. NHS England: Leeds.

19. NHS England. Clinical Pharmacists in General Practice. https://www.england.nhs.uk/commissioning/primary-care-comm/gp-workforce/cp-gp-pilot/. Accessed on 23 July, 2017.

20. NHS England. *Improving medication error incident reporting and learn-ing*. 2014. https://www.england.nhs.uk/wp-content/uploads/2014/03/psa-sup-info-med-error.pdf. Accessed on 23 July, 2017.

21. Parle J, Ennis J. Physician associates: The challenge facing general practice. *Br J Gen Pract*. 2015;65(634):224–5. doi: 10.3399/bjgp15X684685.

22. Drennan VM, Halter M, Joly L, Gage H, Grant RL, Gabe J, Brearley S, Carneiro W, de Lusignan S. Physician associates and GPs in primary care: A comparison. *Br J Gen Pract* 2015;65(634):e344–50.

23. Sinsky CA, Willard-Grace R, Schutzbank AM, Sinsky TA, Margolius D, Bodenheimer T, et al. In search of joy in practice: A report of 23 high-functioning primary care practices. *Ann Fam Med* 2013;11(3):272–8.

24. Goldberg D, Gournay K. *The general practitioner, the psychiatrist, and the burden of mental health care. Maudsley Discussion Paper No. 1*. London: Institute of Psychiatry; 1997.

25. Magnee T, de Beurs DP, de Bakker DH, Verhaak PF. Consultations in gen-eral practices with and without mental health nurses: An observational study from 2010 to 2014. *BMJ Open* 2016;6:e011579.

26. McKinstry B, Walker J, Campbell C, Heaney D, Wyke S. Telephone consultations to manage requests for same-day appointments: A randomised controlled trial in two practices. *Br J Gen Pract* 2002;52(477):306–10.

27. Jiwa M, Mathers N, Campbell M. The effect of GP telephone triage on numbers seeking same-day appointments. *Br J Gen Pract* 2002;52(478):390–1.

28. Holt TA, Fletcher E, Warren F, Richards S, Salisbury C, Calitri R, Green C. Telephone triage systems in UK general practice: Analysis of consultation duration during the index day in a pragmatic randomised controlled trial. *Br J Gen Pract* 2016;66(644):e214–18.

29. Campbell JL, Fletcher E, Britten N, Green C, Holt TA, Lattimer V, Richards DA. Telephone triage for management of same-day consultation requests in general practice (the ESTEEM trial): A cluster randomised controlled trial and cost-consequence analysis. *Lancet.* 2014;384(9957):1859–68.

30. Longman, H. Esteem, Telephones and GP workload. *GP Access.* http://gpaccess.uk/evidence/esteem-telephones-gp-workload/. Accessed on 23 July, 2017.

31. Checkland K, Spooner S. The future of primary care? Reflections on the Primary Care Workforce Commission report. *Br J Gen Pract* 2015;65(639):e633–5. doi: 10.3399/bjgp15X686773.

32. Lewis DM, Naidoo C, Perry J, Watkins J. The Roundhouse: An alternative model for primary care. *Br J Gen Pract* 2016;66(646):e362–4.

33. Heyworth L, Rozenblum R, Burgess JF Jr, Baker E, Meterko M, Prescott D, Neuwirth Z, Simon SR. Influence of shared medical appointments on patient satisfaction: A retrospective 3-year study. *Ann Fam Med* 2014;12(4):324–30.

34. Smith SP, Elias BL. Shared medical appointments: Balancing efficiency with patient satisfaction and outcomes. *Am J Manag Care* 2016;22(7):491–4.

35. Coates J. Shared medical appointments: better by the dozen. *BJGPblog.* 2016. http://bjgpblog.com/2016/06/24/shared-medical-appointments-better-by-the-dozen/. Accessed on 23 July, 2017.

36. Sonala L, Thiel V, Goodwin N, Kodner D. South Devon and Torbay. Proactive case management using the community virtual ward and the Devon Predictive Model. The King's Fund: London. 2013.

37. Bardsley M. Virtual reality: observations from the Nuffield Trust study of Virtual Wards. *Nuffield Trust comment.* 2013. https://www.nuffieldtrust.org.uk/news-item/virtual-reality-observations-from-the-nuffield-trust-study-of-virtual-wards. Accessed on 23 July, 2017.

38. Jeffers H, Baker M. Continuity of care: Still important in modern-day general practice. *Br J Gen Pract* 2016;66(649):396–7.

6

Finding the right career

INTRODUCTION

A newly trained general practitioner (GP) often feels faced with just three career options: a salaried post, a partnership or a period of doing locums. But the choice of career need not be so restricted, and there is an increasing trend towards portfolio careers which allow GPs to combine a variety of roles. This helps to maintain interest and job satisfaction and, by spending regular time away from the ordinary day to day of general practice, many doctors keep their careers feeling fresh.

GPs are in demand in all manner of environments because of the flexibility of their capabilities. This chapter explores some of these different environments, the rewards of working within them and how doctors can find work in these fields.

GP PARTNER

DR. ADAM STATEN
The Red House Surgery, Bletchley

DR. PETER AIRD
East Quay Medical Centre, Bridgwater

General practice in the United Kingdom has long been run on the partnership model, and this continues to be the predominant model for National Health Service (NHS) general practice. For many, the extra administrative and business responsibilities of being a partner seem off-putting, but a partnership offers the opportunity to truly shape the way in which you provide care, gives you independence in how you grow your income and can give the satisfaction of running a small business.

Many GP partners take advantage of these opportunities to work in unconventional ways, take on different roles, and so maintain the interest in general practice that staves off burnout.

What makes being a partner different?

The key difference between a salaried role and a partnership role is the responsibility of running a small business. This brings with it all the financial, administrative and man-management responsibilities that you might expect. Ultimately, your income is dependent on how efficiently and profitably you can run your practice.

The way your surgery runs is determined by you and your partners which gives you control over how you structure your surgeries, what services you offer and which staff you hire. This means you can make your surgery work in a way that suits both you and your patients.

Other aspects of the job

Beyond the management responsibilities of the job, the work you do as a partner will largely depend on what you want to do. As a partner it is between you and your colleagues as to whether you develop a special interest, choose to offer services such as travel clinics or minor surgery or increase your involvement with local or national organisations such as the Clinical Commissioning Group or the British Medical Association.

How to become a partner

Becoming a partner is really about finding a practice with whom you click. You may well be working with the other partners for the rest of your career, so it is important to find colleagues who you are happy to spend a long time working closely with.

The actual mechanics of joining a partnership varies from practice to practice. Some practices require you to 'buy in' to the surgery, which essentially means buying a portion of the physical property of the surgery. Sometimes, this is done with a lump sum, which may require you to take out a loan; alternatively, this can be done gradually by taking a reduced income from the practice over a specified period. Joining a partnership that does not own its own premises is usually a bit more straightforward and does not require buying in.

MY EXPERIENCE: PARTNERING TO AVOID BURNOUT

Dr. Peter Aird
Bridgwater

Since the work of GPs undoubtedly entails the 'long term involvement in emotionally demanding situations', if they are to avoid the emotional, mental and physical exhaustion that is characteristic of burnout, they are going to need a healthy dose of realism. In particular, they must know that they simply cannot meet the constant demands that are placed upon them. To believe otherwise is naïve and, possibly, arrogant, suggesting as it does an inflated sense of one's own power and importance.

Medical science is ever expanding and nobody could possibly keep up with all its advances. Even if one could, each patient's situation is unique and too inordinately complex for science to fully explain. No doctor should imagine, therefore, that he or she could ever be more than a small part of the solution to any of the problems that are presented. As Atul Gawande eloquently explained in the first of his 2014 Reith Lectures, science cannot possibly tell us everything and, consequently, when we fail to meet the needs of others, we do so through our 'necessary fallibility' as much as any deficiency in our own performance.

Working in partnership with others inherently acknowledges one's individual inadequacy and the need for a team approach. Well-organised practices allow the delegation of tasks, both clinical and non-clinical, to those most able to undertake them, be that the chronic disease management undertaken by practice nurses or the annual maximisation of Quality and Outcomes Framework (QOF) points by the effective management of the administration team. Far more than this, however, healthy partnerships allow doctors to lean on one other, to seek advice and guidance, without embarrassment, from colleagues that have differing areas of expertise to their own. Those in healthy partnerships are keen to support their colleagues. They look out for one another and are conscious of those who find themselves overwhelmed. Such partners are willing to take on extra work to lighten the load of another having a bad day and are prepared to respond flexibly to pressures a partner may be experiencing outside of work.

Partnerships also allow partners to take a long-term view. Aware that a medical career is a marathon rather than a sprint, healthy partnerships understand the need for adequate time away from the practice for recuperation and, in addition to protected study time and holidays, factor in the financial cost of periodic extended leave and the occasional sabbatical. Equally, this long-term view will mean older partners would not demand that younger doctors instantly perform at the level of experience they have acquired the moment they join a practice. Rather, they will allow time for them to grow into the role of a GP partner. Likewise, younger doctors will appreciate the wisdom of their older colleagues even if, as they approach retirement, they lack the knowledge of some recent medical advance. Healthy partnerships know medicine is a team sport played over a protracted time, requiring a mix of skills and expertise and, occasionally, temporary substitutions. Think 'Test Match' – not T20!

So what makes a partnership healthy and how can one become so? To support one another as previously suggested, partners need to genuinely care for one another as friends rather than simply existing alongside each other as colleagues. GP partnerships have often been likened to marriages and not without reason. Healthy partnerships are grounded in the commitment that is inherent in partnership and grow as a result of individual partners within them spending time alongside those with whom they go through life and with whom they can honestly acknowledge their weaknesses and struggles. They will not develop where partners stay chained all day to their desk, constantly battling their own struggles all the while oblivious to those being experienced by others. Keeping doors open when not consulting, regularly taking time for informal chat and not neglecting the all-important daily gathering around the coffee machine all serve to build the working friendships that go a long way towards protecting those within those partnerships from burnout. Informal practice meetings over dinner, annual away days and regular social events, all characteristic of healthy partnerships, will go still further.

But there is, I think, an even more fundamental characteristic that healthy partnerships display and which protects those within them from burnout. This might best be described as the partnership ethos – that set of values which define what a partnership considers important and which protects those within the partnership by giving them confidence to stand together against the unrealistic demands of outside forces. Such wisdom comes from those who, through years of experience, have a healthy skepticism for what medicine can do. They know that neither GPs, nor medicine itself, will ever make society as healthy as it desires or demands. They know that constantly striving to prevent the inevitable suffering that is part of being human will exhaust those who try. They also know that one can be a compassionate and caring doctor whilst acknowledging one's inadequacy and uncertainty in that role. They know that to be a doctor is to be flawed and can honestly model that reality to others. Admitting their past errors to younger doctors encourages those young doctors by reassuring them that they are not unique – we all make mistakes sometimes and experience the accompanying painful emotions. Working in healthy partnerships reduces the loneliness one can feel when things go wrong and protects against the burnout that can so easily result. Furthermore, this wisdom, this healthy realism, a feature only of mature stable partnerships, extends beyond the doctors currently in a partnership. It becomes part of the practice consciousness and is handed on to younger partners as they arrive in a practice, encouraging within them a healthy approach to life and work, even as they live and work alongside those nearing the end of their career.

Healthy partnerships are, therefore, necessary to protect doctors against the burnout that must be avoided if they are to continue to like their patients and enjoy trying to do their best for them. The support such partnerships provide, and the realism they engender, allows GPs to be realistic with their patients and thereby help them, in turn, to be realistic about what medicine has to offer them and society as a whole. All this serves to mitigate against the burden of demand that GPs can feel is placed upon them. As such, rather than being seen as something entered into with trepidation, a GP partnership should be something that is desired and valued highly, seen as the essential it is for healthy GPs and, consequently, a healthy practice population.

THE REMOTE AND RURAL GP

DR. KATE DAWSON

Benbecula Medical Practice, Outer Hebrides

I am a GP in Benbecula, one of the islands in the Outer Hebrides. I have been working here for more than 25 years. Working in a rural environment allows me to stay in one of the loveliest parts of Britain, in a small and effective team, with lots of opportunity for personal growth, extended roles, responsibility and achievement. My family and I are also intrinsic to the community.

What makes rural general practice different?

The key difference between rural, remote and island practice and that of an urban GP is geographical access to resources. We work miles away from district and rural general hospitals. Getting a CT scan may involve major logistics, and visiting a specialist can result in journeys of hundreds of miles, with flights and ferries, hotel costs and hospital canteen food.

This distance from advanced services means that rural GPs generally offer extended services, often providing a significant contribution to local out of hours arrangements, supplementing specialist services or being available for emergencies and pre-hospital care. I find considerable satisfaction in designing realistic goals of care for patients that consider a desire to be treated within the rural community. This can mean that we undertake clinical responsibility that would not be considered in an urban setting. This problem solving can include setting up videolink clinical reviews, monitoring blood gases and delivering regular infusions and transfusions in a community setting.

Teamwork with other health and social care professionals is also very close and bespoke. We are generally on first-name terms with members of the health and social care team and meet regularly for clinical reviews. Because we are in a small health board, we have great access to our local consultants; we often phone them up for advice about how to avoid an admission, or whether a referral is required. They sometimes visit the area to undertake clinics, and this is a great opportunity to arrange training.

One significant part of living in a very remote area is access to the outdoor, unbuilt environment. This is part of our work and our recreation and shapes the lives of our patients, and the planning of our services. Many remote and rural GPs are attracted to the islands because they are seeking places to kayak, dive, windsurf, sail, climb, hike and explore.

Rural practitioners work and live in small communities, patients do not have much choice about which practice they attend and GPs cannot live away from their patients. The consequence of this is that a rural GP is a significant figure in their community, for better or for worse. We are accountable to the people that we live amongst, and our ethical and moral values are visible and must be sound.

Other aspects of the job

By being remote, rural general practice runs the risk of being overlooked. Rural practitioners have to work hard to maintain their profile and their high standards.

Networking is an important facet of the life of a rural GP. Distance means that attending traditional lunchtime educational events and meetings is impractical. We use videoconferencing and web-streaming to access education, and to attend meetings. Social media such as Twitter, Facebook and Slack allow us to keep in contact with other rural GPs. Issues such as recruitment, role development, safe clinical pathways and education are all explored in our virtual community. Being part of a group of interested, talented professionals with high academic, ethical and humanitarian standards is very rewarding.

The Royal College of General Practitioners (RCGP) has a rural forum which aims to ensure that new policies are rural proof and that access to consultation is fair. They have a remit to represent rural practitioners, supporting the development of professional networks and promoting rural practice as an exhilarating and professionally fulfilling career.

The Rural GP Association of Scotland runs an annual conference and provides support to students interested in rural general practice and WONCA has a rural branch, the WONCA Working Party on Rural Practice, where ideas and good practice are shared at an international level.

Rural practitioners also have a big role to play in training the next generation. Ironically, some practices are deemed too small to give students enough clinical contact, but the high-intensity, detailed and patient-centred opportunities in rural practice can be very high value. Most rural practices are highly sought-after placements for medical students and junior doctors.

We have a role in supporting rural applicants into medical careers, mentoring school pupils, coaching medical students, providing taster sessions for foundation year 1 and 2 doctors, and providing training placements for would-be rural GPs. One of the best aspects of rural practice is the need to innovate to improve care for our communities. There is no one in a centre of excellence who knows more about the barriers to accessing standard care, and no one who is better placed to overcome those barriers. Through innovation, new higher standards of care can be created.

Career options in rural general practice

Rural GPs have the opportunity to shape their roles according to the physical and clinical environment in which they operate.

The areas where we practice may include mountains, the oceans, contrasts in weather or large areas crossed by major transport routes. Some GPs undertake work with the coastguard, join mountain rescue teams, or provide medical cover with research and rescue helicopters or clinical support to military bases.

In the smaller, more remote health boards, the resources offered by secondary care are often run through obligate clinical networks. These are greatly enhanced by GPs with additional skills. The chance to work part-time in general practice and part-time in a specialty allows rural GPs the reward of extending their roles. I work in a dermatology clinic as well as in primary care, and I know other rural GPs who also provide palliative care, community child health, gynaecology, sexual health clinics, care of the elderly and accident & emergency department (A&E) sessions. One of my partners is the local lead for major incident planning, and we practice with other emergency services in an annual major incident drill.

Community hospitals

Medical care in community hospitals is normally led by GPs. The range of services provided varies enormously, but can include A&E facilities, usually staffed by emergency nurse practitioners, supported by GPs. Patients with severe trauma need to be stabilised and acute medical conditions such as myocardial infarction, stroke and exacerbations of chronic obstructive pulmonary disease (COPD) or asthma can all be effectively managed in this setting.

The sick child can provide particular challenges. Patients requiring specialist care or investigation need to be transferred after stabilisation. Midwife-led maternity services, often with GP support, allow low-risk births to take place in the community. Rehabilitation, if appropriate occupational therapy and physiotherapy services are available, can be delivered effectively in community hospitals. Palliative care facilities are particularly important to allow people to die in comfort and dignity within their own community.

BECOMING A RURAL GP

Dr. Catherine Brown

Shetland Islands

Having had a semi-rural upbringing in the north of Scotland, I always had a desire to want to return to the rural environment and, whilst at medical school, I undertook a 3-month placement in rural General Practice in Perthshire. I found the placement inspirational, affording me truly unique and rich clinical experiences.

I undertook my GP training on the Scottish Rural Track GP Training Programme. The training offered was broad based and focussed on producing rural generalists.

My first year was spent working at the Gilbert Bain Hospital in Lerwick, doing medicine, surgery, A&E and everything in between. There were no registrars, and so there was increased clinical responsibility – which I found very rewarding. We worked closely with nursing staff and Consultant colleagues, and I really enjoyed this teamwork.

The remainder of my training was spent between other hospital specialties and general practice. In Shetland we have adopted a hub-and-spoke model within general practice training, with trainees spending most of their time at Lerwick Health Centre (Lerwick being the main town with a practice list size of approximately 9000 patients).

For several weeks of the year, trainees head out to single-handed practices to get more of an appreciation of how this practice differs. I enjoyed the contrast, in particular the continuity of care that can be offered within the smaller practices and the excitement of out of hours work.

Part of the Rural Track training scheme included a funded BASICS, Pre-Hospital Emergency Care Course, which has certainly helped me feel better prepared for dealing with providing health care in the pre-hospital environment.

The rural fellowship

NHS Education for Scotland has recognised that being a rural GP requires additional skills and runs a rural GP fellowship year for qualified GPs. The training and mentoring provided during the year develop the skills of GPs so that they can step into a rural GP role with confidence.

The rural fellowship posts come in two flavours: the standard fellowship, which is primarily practice based, and a more acute version, often based in acute care community hospitals, providing a blend of general practice and some more acute medicine, including A&E and out of hours.

Each fellow is based in a rural practice or acute community hospital with a local mentor. The year includes 13 weeks of protected training time which includes courses, residential teaching sessions and placements to meet learning needs. There is a financial allowance to support the learning program, which is designed to meet each fellow's learning needs. A quarter of the year should be spent at the base practice, and the rest of the year is spent on service delivery as required by the host health board. This could include working in other remote practices, or joining the out-of-hours rota.

MY EXPERIENCE

Dr. Kate Dawson
Outer Hebrides

Benbecula and the Uists form part of the Western Isles. The islands are located 40 miles off the northwest coast of Scotland, 130 miles long from the Butt of Lewis in the north to the Isle of Barra in the south. The population of the Western Isles is approximately 26,500, spread over 280 townships.

Around 22% of the population are more than 65 years old, proportionately one of the most elderly populations in Scotland.

There are three practices on the three main islands; I am a partner at Benbecula Medical Practice, which is a dispensing practice based on the central island. In addition to providing primary care services, we also provide medical cover to St. Kilda, the rocket range and the airport.

After I joined the practice, we took on the contract to provide medical cover to the island community hospital. The community hospital has changed quite a lot over time. In the 1960s, the hospital had surgical and anaesthetic support, which our practice took over in the 1990s, with GPs who were also trained as surgeons and anaesthetists. These skills are now no longer widely available in the GP community, but one of my GP colleagues has a background in anaesthetics and emergency medicine, making him a very valuable resource.

In that time, the hospital has moved to a new building, and now has 16 beds, rising to 20 beds when there is additional pressure. The inpatient beds are used to provide acute medical care for patients that either do not need to be airlifted to another hospital, or whose ceiling of care is for local care only. This can include acute medical care such as pneumonia and exacerbation of COPD, or rehabilitation after orthopaedic surgery.

We also provide acute assessment and A&E services. Because we are on an island, we are a non-bypass community hospital, providing services for acute coronary syndrome, strokes, trauma, acute abdominal pain and similar presentations. We are supported by a team of nurses with extended clinical skills. We have a minilab that can undertake a range of near-patient tests and a small x-ray department that provides a service during the day, with films being uploaded onto PACS so that we can get external advice. There is also a weekly visiting scan clinic.

Patients who exceed the capacity of our hospital are airlifted to definitive places of care. The support of the Emergency Medical Retrieval Service and ScotStar make the air transport of our more unwell patients much safer, and they also provide excellent remote management support.

Over the past few years, we have developed a number of clinical pathways and guidance tools to help us provide consistently high-quality clinical care even though we are not experts, nor do we see these presentations as often as an acute medical unit.

Conclusions

The advantages of rural medicine include the huge satisfaction of providing holistic, traditional general practice, integrated into the community, and developing and maintaining a wide range of skills. The rural environment is wonderful for raising families, with small and generally excellent schools. The opportunities for recreation outside work are amazing – the wilderness is right up against the garden fence.

There are challenges. Without effort, professional isolation can be a burden and there are on-call commitments and times of high stress, coupled with a potential lack of privacy and anonymity. We are rural generalists, working in systems where the volume of patients may be lower than in the urban setting but the intensity and the depth of the clinical experience is unmatched. It is an honour to be a GP working in a rural community.

THE OVERSEAS GP

DR. TIM SENIOR

Tharawal Aboriginal Corporation, Airds, NSW Australia

One of the privileges of a medical degree is that doctors are respected and able to get work in most countries around the world. While it can be a wonderful escapist fantasy, fuelled by recruitment advertisement images of pristine beaches and diving adventures, the reality can be a little different. Uprooting yourself, and perhaps your family, from familiar surroundings and friends is not easy, but with the right planning and a little flexibility it can be the best move you ever make.

What makes overseas general practice different?

There is only one thing that can be guaranteed about working as a GP overseas: it will be different. The NHS is a unique institution, and working in another country will expose you to another way of running a health system, with varying degrees of success, each with its own rewards and frustrations. In some places, you may have easy access to investigations without waiting lists, while in others you might be working under a tree with a limited supply of simple medications.

The principles of your general practice work will be the same wherever you are, in providing first contact and ongoing care for people who come to see you. The organisation of this will make your work very different. In most countries, you will not have a defined population of patients, and you may not have particularly good information technology. You may find that hospitals and specialists are the main focus of the system. The mechanics of referrals, requests for investigations, allied health, psychology, how medications are provided, and the way all of these are funded will undoubtedly be different, and a little tedious to learn.

Many countries put restrictions on where you are allowed to work, and you may find yourself only allowed to work in areas not well served by home-grown doctors. Many of these places are beautiful, but you may be a long way from cities, schools, sources of work for partners or cultural activities. For many of us raised in the United Kingdom, it can be difficult to appreciate how big many other countries are.

There will be all sorts of specifics to get your head around about visa requirements, registration requirements (even with the possibility of having to do more exams) and continuing professional development requirements, although there will usually be agencies that are able to guide you around these multiple labyrinths. Whatever the health system, in many places around the world, the services you are able to offer may be limited by the patients' ability to pay. For those of us brought up in the NHS that can be a frustrating experience.

To a varying degree, there will be language differences to overcome, some just subtle variations of English and some where you will be practicing with translators in your second language. The cultural norms will be different, even if you are working in the Anglosphere. These differences are very difficult to prepare for, and the best way to manage them is to immerse yourself whole-heartedly, find local people prepared to guide you and think hard. In many Anglophone countries, culture will extend to understanding something of the local indigenous cultures, too, as these will be different to the mainstream cultures, and you are likely to be at the forefront of their health problems. These cultural norms may also extend to the way GPs are viewed. Most places will be very grateful to have a new doctor in their community, but there are countries where they might wish you were a 'clever' brain surgeon, rather than 'just a GP'.

Other aspects of the job

In countries such as Australia and Canada, you are often required to work in a rural area, and the scope of practice is frequently wider than you might be used to. GPs often provide acute emergency care; obstetric, anaesthetic or surgical care; and manage inpatients, as well as regular general practice work. In other places you will require higher level skills in mental health or public health. Training will often be available to update your skills in these areas if required.

As well as clinical care, there will be other responsibilities that come with your role. Administrative tasks are complained about wherever you work and may not be remunerated. There may be good opportunities for managerial and leadership roles within your practice or in the local area. You may be called on to provide public health advice. In most places there will be the opportunity for teaching junior doctors, medical students and other health professionals. Some countries may also offer opportunities for research.

Your work will also depend on your employment context. In some countries, you will be running a business, maybe as a contractor. Alternatively, you might be employed, either by government, a private company, a philanthropic organisa-tion or a co-operative. This may alter your work, in the way you are expected (or not!) to provide business or advocacy expertise in the course of your work.

Many opportunities available depend on the health system in the country in which you are working. Many countries have a less well-developed primary care system, and GPs may be seen as the poor (in all senses of the word) cousin of proper specialist doctors. Doctors in just about every country are highly sought after and highly regarded, though, so there are often opportunities to construct a career of your choosing.

Career options in overseas general practice

Working as a GP overseas can be as flexible as you want it to be. You will often have the chance of part-time clinical work, with the remainder filled by academic, educational, management or leadership roles. In some places the formal organ-isational structures, such as public health, government or professional bodies, may be well established and provide opportunities for non-clinical (but perhaps unpaid) work. There are likely to be entrepreneurial opportunities in most places, too, business opportunities for patient care, education or consultancy work.

For the most part, there will not be a clearly defined career structure. Formal employment in an academic institution may have opportunities for a career pathway, but beyond buying into a practice and ongoing professional education, many GPs determine their own pathways. This can lead to a feeling of being stuck, but it can also create a sense of freedom or opportunity about the future without a predetermined pathway.

How to become an overseas GP

The logistics of working in another country can be complex, and it is worth seeking advice early. Social media makes it easier than ever before to have informal conversations with local doctors, or those who have already made the journey before you, and their advice will be invaluable.

If you have not completed your GP training, your options will be more limited, but there are opportunities. It may be possible to have temporary overseas work accredited towards your training, but this should be confirmed beforehand. The RCGP International offers a limited number of opportunities for GPs in training and those in their first 5 years. However, outside these official programs, in some countries it may be difficult to complete your training overseas, and you may find you have to start again.

Once fully qualified, the Membership of the Royal College of General Practitioners (MRCGP) qualification is highly regarded and in many countries is recognised as a GP qualification, allowing you to work without much further assessment. In some places, however, you may need to sit an exam or have some other assessment of your skills. Other qualifications will be very useful in demonstrating higher skills in clinical areas, such as paediatrics, obstetrics or anaesthetics, or in non-clinical areas, such as public health, medical education or medical administration.

Along with your medical degree and higher medical qualifications, each country has separate requirements for registration, immigration and perhaps for payment through government or private insurance programs. You will need to get a certificate of good standing from the General Medical Council (GMC), and overseas registration authorities may examine your disciplinary record quite closely, after examples in several countries of this not being done well.

Immigration requirements mean you have to ensure that the visa you are on allows you to work, and there may be other restrictions on how long you can work or where you can live or travel. Similarly, the differences in health systems and payment arrangements, in conjunction with workforce policies, can ensure that your options about where you can work in your chosen country may be limited.

It is also important to look at your medical indemnity. Your UK medical indemnity is unlikely to cover you overseas, except perhaps for volunteer or humanitarian work, and you will need to find a local insurer.

Finding a job might be done through word of mouth, or through recruitment and locum agencies.

MY EXPERIENCE

Dr. Tim Senior
NSW Australia

My own example of coming to Australia serves to illustrate the combination of planning, opportunities and sheer luck that characterise much of working overseas.

My first job as a GP in Australia was in Alice Springs, right in the middle of Australia, 1000 miles away from the nearest tertiary referral centres. Work in Australia as an international medical graduate will restrict you to more out-of-the-way places that struggle to recruit, but these can also be some of the more fascinating places to work. Much is made of the procedural skills, such as anaesthetics or obstetrics, required in many remote and rural areas, but there are certainly useful roles for GPs without those skills, too.

Because I was married to an Australian I had permanent residency. Many GPs working in Australia will have specific work visas and be temporary residents, and at the time of writing some of these visas are the subject of political discussion.

In Alice Springs I also had the opportunity to do fly-in fly-out clinics every fortnight to a remote Aboriginal community 400 km south of town, which was a completely different experience to anything I had done up to that point. While I was young and relatively inexperienced, the core skills of general practice allowed me to manage safely, and to improve.

A year in Alice Springs showed up some of the changing challenges that can combine overseas. A combination of newborn twins and lack of close family support meant a move away to be closer to family in the outskirts of one of Australia's big cities. I lined up work in a general practice which fell through because of government restrictions on the location of practices I was allowed to work in. After a panicky few months, I managed to get work as a medical educator (the Australian equivalent of a GP Tutor) on the GP Training Program. The restrictions on location do not apply to academic non-clinical work.

A few months after that I asked about work in a local Aboriginal Community Controlled Health Service. This combination effectively found me my niche in Australian medicine. I have continued my clinical work in Aboriginal and Torres Strait Islander health and taken opportunities that arise from this to work in areas of education and policy with the Royal Australian College of General Practitioners and to write on these for various publications. It is this combination of work that has successfully enabled me to avoid burnout in a career often thought of as a challenging area in which to work.

My career was not planned from the start, though I was clear about the sort of work that I was most interested in. It is this combination of career goals with problem solving and flexibility – all attributes required for general practice – that allows for successful wellbeing from working overseas.

Conclusions

Overseas work can give rise to new opportunities and new experiences. There can be a myriad of bureaucratic hoops to jump through, involving visas, medical registration, insurance and registration with government and private insurance payment systems. However, a combination of good research and planning your trip, together with the ability to be flexible, will enable you to make the most of work in another country and enhance your own wellbeing.

THE MILITARY GP

DR. ADAM STATEN

The Red House Surgery, Bletchley

GPs are the backbone of the Defence Medical Services which provide health care for the military, and unlike military secondary care consultants who are usually embedded within NHS hospitals, military GPs operate entirely within the military system.

All units within the armed forces, from engineer regiments to naval battleships, have GPs attached to them to provide care for our soldiers, sailors and aircrew. These GPs need to have a specific set of skills to deal with the unique challenges that military life can present, and they are not only doctors but are also military officers who take on all the responsibilities that this entails. General practice in the forces offers a career that is truly both military and medical.

What makes military general practice different?

The most obvious difference between military general practice and its NHS counterpart is the patient population that it serves. The service population is aged almost entirely between 18 and 55 and is still predominantly male so there is little or no paediatrics, no geriatrics, and far less obstetrics and gynaecology than in civilian practice. This population is also pre-screened so that, at least on enlistment, the population is relatively free from illness and disease.

Furthermore, if a serviceman or woman develops a chronic illness, it is often incompatible with on-going military service. Any condition that is likely to become unstable if treatment is interrupted, such as epilepsy or type 1 diabetes, is likely to lead to discharge from the forces and whilst other chronic conditions, such as hypertension or hypothyroidism, may be suitable for continued service, there is little chronic disease management in the military.

Military doctors are most occupied with a range of other conditions that usually form a smaller part of the NHS workload. As you might expect, there is a great deal of musculoskeletal medicine within the military. In this respect servicemen and women are seen as professional athletes whose livelihoods, and very often whose lives, depend on the good functioning of their bodies. Therefore, provision for musculoskeletal problems is excellent and GPs are central to the assessment and management of them.

There is also a relatively large amount of tropical medicine within the military. With personnel travelling worldwide, GPs are involved both with preparing service personnel for travel and for remaining alert to the array of peculiar illnesses that people may present with whilst away or once back at home.

Occupational medicine is a big issue within the armed forces. Although there is a cadre of military doctors devoted to occupational medicine, the bulk of this work falls to GPs who are responsible for establishing to what extent illness and injury stop soldiers, sailors and aircrew from performing their duty; for how long this will be the case; and whether this needs to be referred onto the occupational health specialists. Consequently, military doctors are given a great deal of training in this area.

The skill set that military GPs possess that is probably most alien to an NHS GP is that required to deal with trauma, both on and off the battlefield. A military GP is expected to be able to deal with the immediate aftermath of all manner of major trauma including gunshot wounds, traumatic amputations, burns and road traffic accidents. As such they are highly trained, and often highly experienced, in haemorrhage control, airway management and a range of other skills that are usually the preserve of trauma specialists and paramedics in civilian medicine.

Because of the diversity of functions within the military there is a wide array of specialist areas in which GPs can work including aviation medicine, sports and rehabilitation medicine, expedition medicine, dive medicine or mountain medicine. The armed forces treasure training and will pay for their doctors to be trained in almost anything if a sound case can be made to justify the expense.

Other aspects of the job

A military doctor is an officer embedded within the working world of the unit he or she is serving with. This means that the doctor, or medical officer, is expected to take on non-medical responsibilities which might include being the duty officer who deals with any problems that crop up on base, organising entertainments in the officer's mess or taking charge of organising sports within the unit.

Military GPs are intimately involved in planning big military exercises, both at home and overseas, and in planning casualty evacuation strategies and the deployment of medical assets during active, war-fighting operations. They are also involved with the planning and execution of military responses to humanitarian crises such as earthquakes and famine.

For prolonged operations the medical officer will also have to create plans to deal with mass casualties; plans for the quarantine and treatment of contagious disease; and environmental health plans to prevent infectious diseases, such as diarrhoeal illness and malaria, taking hold in the first place.

Career options in the military

Increasingly, the three branches of the armed forces work collaboratively in providing medical care. A naval medical officer was not an uncommon sight in landlocked Afghanistan, and it is not unheard of for an army doctor to be found aboard a naval vessel. However, the roles of the three forces are still fairly separate, so medical careers within each force can be quite different.

As an army GP you may find yourself supporting armoured units operating in armoured vehicles, supporting the infantry in ground-based operations or attached to engineer or logistics units responsible for the smooth running of an operation or exercise. During the recent conflicts in Iraq and Afghanistan, GPs with specialist pre-hospital emergency medicine skills were also used aboard the emergency helicopters that responded to battlefield casualties.

Naval GPs are responsible for the day-to-day primary health care of sailors whilst they are on shore and will then go to sea with their units. Aboard a ship a naval GP may run a small sick bay where sailors can be bedded down and treated for more serious conditions without the need to fly them off to dry land. GPs are also attached to submarine crews with the responsibility of making sure that the crew is in tip-top physical shape before they, and their doctor, disappear beneath the waves. Evacuating sick patients from a top secret submarine that is never supposed to surface provides quite a challenge and is best avoided if possible.

GPs within the Royal Air Force receive extra training in aviation medicine. They are also expected to be able to respond to aircraft emergencies and crashes that may occur on the station on which they are serving. The aeromedical evacuation of wounded servicemen from warzones is another area in which Royal Air Force GPs are involved.

In all three services, there are opportunities to develop special interests, engage in research and take roles in staff and command, managing the structure and running of the medical services whilst sacrificing patient contact.

How to become a military GP

Many GPs in the military sign up to the services whilst at university and undertake their vocational training under the auspices of the defence medical deanery. However, there are opportunities to join the services after training. Like the NHS, the armed forces are short of GPs; therefore, all three services actively recruit fully trained GPs and often offer a financial incentive to join.

Once a GP has enlisted, he or she then goes through a period of military training at one of the forces colleges where instruction is provided in military skills alongside other professionally qualified officers such as lawyers and chaplains. Traditionally, these were 4-week crash courses in marching, polishing and drinking port, known as 'tarts and vicars courses', but in response to the frontline involvement of doctors in Afghanistan and Iraq, these courses were extended and intensified so that doctors could conduct themselves safely in warzones.

The armed forces in the modern era are shifting to an increasing reliance on reserve personnel, and this is good news for any doctor wishing to get involved with the military without devoting themselves entirely to the forces. With a paid commitment of as little of 27 days a year, the reserve forces offer the opportunity to participate in all aspects of military life whilst maintaining a life in the civilian world.

MY EXPERIENCE

Dr. Adam Staten
Bletchley

I served in the Nahr-e Saraj and Nad-e Ali districts of Helmand province, Afghanistan, between March and October 2012. Operations in Helmand were run on a 'hub-and-spoke model'. At the centre sat Camp Bastion where a large hospital was located; around this were 'main operating bases' where there might be several GPs located together, and around these were the Patrol Bases which either had a GP or a more junior 'General Duties Medical Officer' supporting a population of between 100 and 200 soldiers.

Helmand was a harsh environment. During the summer temperatures reached 50°C, and soldiers patrolled wearing armour and carrying equipment that often weighed in excess of 60 kg. The most feared enemy threat was the 'improvised explosive device' which was responsible for numerous deaths and for many soldiers suffering life-changing injuries, but there were also threats from snipers, grenade attacks, mortar fire and the ubiquitous AK-47. It was a frightening place.

Helmand posed particular medical threats as well. 'Helmand fever' was a blanket term used for an assorted array of parasitic, febrile illnesses that included malaria and tick typhus, which popped up occasionally, and there was also the potential for spider and snake bites. But by far the most common problem was simple diarrhoea and vomiting. Sanitation was difficult, and people were living in very close proximity to one another. Diarrhoea and vomiting bugs could spread like wildfire through a camp and render the entire unit completely unable to do its duty.

As a medical officer there were long periods of boredom dealing with sprained ankles and infected insect bites, but these were interspersed with episodes of frank terror. I spent the majority of my time within the relative safety of the patrol base, but for big or prolonged operations I would go out on the ground, either on foot or in armoured vehicles, to best position myself to receive casualties who would be brought back to me from the fighting on stretchers or on quad-bike trailers. I would look after these soldiers until the helicopter mounted 'medical emergency response team' swooped gloriously out of the sky.

Whilst in camp I provided medical care for a platoon of soldiers from the Afghan Army, and I provided training both for our soldiers and the Afghans in how to deal with battlefield injuries. Beyond my medical duties I spent many long hours manning the radios at nighttime and helping to plan the casualty evacuation plans for operations.

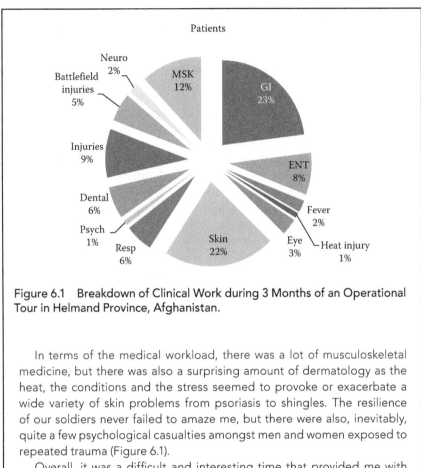

Figure 6.1   Breakdown of Clinical Work during 3 Months of an Operational Tour in Helmand Province, Afghanistan.

In terms of the medical workload, there was a lot of musculoskeletal medicine, but there was also a surprising amount of dermatology as the heat, the conditions and the stress seemed to provoke or exacerbate a wide variety of skin problems from psoriasis to shingles. The resilience of our soldiers never failed to amaze me, but there were also, inevitably, quite a few psychological casualties amongst men and women exposed to repeated trauma (Figure 6.1).

Overall, it was a difficult and interesting time that provided me with experiences that would simply not have been open to me in civilian practice.

Conclusions

Life as a military GP can be exciting, challenging and occasionally dangerous. The armed forces offer the chance for an entirely different career within general practice, with opportunities to practice in austere and hostile environments, develop unusual special interests, travel and take on command responsibilities.

Furthermore, the increasing reliance of the forces on reserve personnel means that it need not be an all-or-nothing commitment; instead, it can provide regular, paid periods of respite from the day to day of NHS general practice.

THE ENTREPRENEURIAL GP

DR. KNUT SCHROEDER

Founder and Director, Expert Self Care Ltd

Being an entrepreneurial GP can be an exciting, stimulating and rewarding adventure. Opportunities for flexible career structures and a comparatively good income allow GPs to set up new businesses without having to lose their steady pay cheque or give up the day job. But while many GPs have managed to convert their innovative ideas into thriving ventures, their journey to success has often been challenging and tough – requiring hard work, dedication and self-motivation.

Setting up a social enterprise – a business or organisation that applies commercial strategies to improve human wellbeing – may be an approach that suits GPs well, because it is not only concerned with creating profits for yourself and other shareholders but also aims to maximise social impact and benefit society.

What makes entrepreneurial general practice different?

Working as a GP in the NHS is largely about providing individual patient care as an independent contractor. As an entrepreneurial GP, the focus of the work shifts from caring for individual patients to creating products for the wider population or other businesses, including other general practices. Examples of enterprises run by GPs include providing clinical services for other practices, building and renting out property for health purposes, developing new medical devices, delivering new and innovative services to the NHS or individual patients, and creating information technology (IT) solutions.

Much of the work of NHS GPs is reactive, such as meeting patient needs, dealing with test results or supporting the practice team in their daily work. In addition, GPs have to fulfil contractual obligations. In contrast, setting up a new business and being entrepreneurial requires a more proactive approach guided by a wider vision and sustained by generating and testing ideas. This involves taking risks, offset by the belief that the investment in terms of time and money will pay off in the future. It seems that many GPs become entrepreneurs because they feel intrinsically motivated to make a difference to people's lives and because they enjoy it, not because they are in it for the money.

Depending on the type of business and the product, setting up a new business will need internal or external funding. This may mean that GP entrepreneurs need to use personal savings, take up a bank loan, apply for grants or obtain investment from sponsors or investors to finance their new venture. Creating a concise and clear business plan and being realistic about financial projections can help maintain sufficient cash-flow, which is essential for making your business viable and sustainable in the long run.

Becoming an entrepreneur also involves learning new skills around starting and running a business, developing products or services, planning and managing projects, funding, marketing, networking, securing and overseeing finances, dealing with different types of stakeholders and customers and understanding the legal aspects of creating and running an enterprise. For people new to business, plenty of support is widely available – from business blogs, books and courses to websites and online videos. Many GPs starting a new business already have experience in recruiting and managing teams, which is useful for creating and leading a team as part of a new business venture.

One of the key differences between NHS work and being an entrepreneur is the comparative freedom that the latter allows. While NHS GPs largely work within given frameworks such as the QOF and need to fulfil requirements set by the CQC, entrepreneurial GPs can focus on creating something that other people or organisations need or want – and get paid for it. While the demands of running your own business can be high, being your own boss, having the freedom to make high-level decisions quickly and being able to work flexibly can provide high job satisfaction. Creating new and innovative solutions for problems that are real 'pain-points' for patients, fellow health professionals or the wider health sector can also be stimulating and rewarding.

Other aspects of the job

Being a successful GP entrepreneur also involves building new relationships with other people and establishing networks that include fellow entrepreneurs, experts, potential and existing customers and other professionals. The concept of 'networking' may not come naturally to some GPs, but meeting and talking with new people, sharing experiences with them and providing mutual support often leads to new friendships and inspiring experiences that enrich their lives. Useful opportunities for networking include conferences and professional events, followed up by emails, phone calls or connecting via social media (such as Twitter).

Setting up a new business and developing a product or service can have other benefits and may provide new opportunities. For example, being seen as an 'expert' in a certain area may lead to invitations to speak at conferences and other events, write blog posts or book chapters or engage in media interviews.

Becoming an entrepreneur may take up more of your time than you had thought. Sometimes the only way to get work done will be to get up earlier in the morning, work into the night or on weekends or stop other non-essential activities and pastimes. Effective time management can help with maintaining a healthy balance between the 'day-job', family life, hobbies and other commitments. Various online tools are available to help manage your time, for example, by storing and sharing your files and resources, or by helping you communicate with your team.

Career options in entrepreneurial general practice

There is no one way of becoming an entrepreneurial GP and starting your own business, and there are no fixed career structures. But there are almost limitless opportunities. One of the first things to decide will be whether you want to start a business venture within or outside your traditional GP role.

Working from within a partnership may provide some protection, especially when things become difficult, because you may share some or all of the risks with your partners. But getting partners on board and involved with your business venture and getting enough protected time to move your new venture forward is not always easy.

If you decide to go it alone and become your own 'stand-alone' entrepreneur, it is worth thinking about how much time and other resources you need to start and run your new business. An important consideration will be to get a feeling for how likely your new business and your new product are to succeed. Creating at least a rough business plan and getting early feedback can help estimate the expected benefits and risks, especially if getting feedback involves people who would be potential customers or users.

How to become an entrepreneurial GP

Leaving general practice altogether and becoming a full-time entrepreneur can be risky, especially if you have a mortgage and a family to maintain. But there is another way: by devoting only a certain amount of time to your new business venture and continuing your GP work, you can become an entrepreneur and be your own boss while keeping risks manageable.

If you are prepared to learn as you go along, you do not need any prior business experience to become a successful entrepreneur. As a GP you already have many of the abilities and the expertise needed for setting up a business, such as communication skills, leading a team, making quick decisions and dealing with uncertainty. A learning needs analysis may help you identify your business-specific training needs, many of which can be addressed by reading around relevant subjects, enrolling in online courses and attending local business training sessions.

Having a good business idea will be key. If you work to your strengths and create a product or service that is related to general practice or that uses any other personal skills or prior experience that you have (such as teaching, training or IT), this puts you at an immediate advantage.

To increase the chances of success, your product should solve a problem, create a new solution or make a difference to people's lives or to organisations – perhaps by creating time for people, saving them money, or by making their life or work easier. Other important issues to consider are the potential size of your market (locally, regionally, nationally or even globally), your profit margins (the amount by which your revenue exceeds your costs) and how you will make your customers aware of your product (marketing and promotion).

Speaking with your accountant early on about your business idea and getting legal advice can help you avoid costly pitfalls, especially if you are about to create a new brand, need to write and sign contracts or want to develop a product, when, for instance, protecting your intellectual property rights may become an issue.

MY EXPERIENCE

Dr. Knut Schroeder
Expert Self Care Ltd

After working as an academic GP for a few years, I became a part-time (six sessions) GP Partner in 2005. My days off I spent either with my family or on other projects – especially projects that involved writing for GPs or patients. I also developed an interest in self-care.

In 2012 a colleague working in student health asked me if I could write a health information book for young people who have left home and have started to go to university. This seemed a good idea, but when I presented it to some students to get their feedback, they said they would not be interested in a book. Instead, they said they would prefer it if we could develop an app for them instead.

At the time, I did not own a smartphone and had no real concept of the usefulness of apps, so I started doing some research. It quickly became clear to me that health information apps had great potential and that there was a gap in the market – and that creating a smartphone app seemed achievable.

Having made the decision to go ahead, we decided to create a social enterprise and register it as a limited company. To help us ensure that the information on the app was going to be reliable, we started working towards NHS England Information Standard certification, which we were awarded in 2014.

Because I was not an expert in student health, I involved the clinical team of the University of Bristol Students' Health Service in creating the content for this app. To ensure that the app addressed the needs of students, we also assembled a student panel that was more than 25 strong, whose input proved invaluable, especially when it came to testing our (often wrong) assumptions. We also recruited a local app developer, a graphic designer and a web designer.

Setting up this new venture has been exciting and rewarding, although it required a lot of my time and energy. Keeping my clinical work going and taking a 'lean' approach to setting up the business allowed me to manage risks carefully, even if this meant that developing the app took a bit longer.

Key lessons that I have learned are to always test my assumptions with potential users or customers, to involve users and experts right from the start and to choose my team carefully, because it really helps if you get on well and work with people who are good at what they do.

The app was finally launched in June 2016, but the initial pick-up was much slower than expected. But sustained marketing efforts helped us generate interest in the app and gave it some traction. I enjoy being my own boss and the freedom that comes with it while still doing clinical work as a locum GP. It seems fair to say though that putting in the hours and 'keeping going' can be a challenge.

Conclusions

Becoming an entrepreneurial GP can be fun and rewarding, but it is not for everyone. GPs wanting to set up their own business are in a privileged position because they are likely to have some choice over their working patterns. Being a GP entrepreneur can complement your clinical work and family life – but it can be tough and sometimes even lonely. Important ingredients to success are building a supportive network, working with people you like and getting early and regular feedback on your ideas.

Useful further reading, links and resources

Business for Punks by James Watt. Portfolio Penguin, 2015.
Social Enterprise UK: http://www.socialenterprise.org.uk/
The Lean Startup by Eric Ries. Crown Publishing Group, 2011.
Running a limited company: https://www.gov.uk/running-a-limited-company
Business and self-employed: https://www.gov.uk/browse/business
The 10% Entrepreneur: Live Your Startup Dream Without Quitting Your Day
    Job by Patrick J McGuinness. Portfolio, 2016.

THE HUMANITARIAN GP

DR. REBECCA FARRINGTON

GPwSI in Refugee Health, Clinical Lecturer, University of Manchester

A 'humanitarian' is defined as 'one who is devoted to the promotion of human welfare and the advancement of social reform' or a 'person who works to make other people's lives better'. I am sure all GPs will recognise humanitarianism in their roles wherever they work. We all have a patient-centred focus and require a holistic approach. We are motivated first and foremost by improving the wellbeing of our patients, regardless of context.

The differences in my role as a GP for people seeking asylum are the lack of resources available to the patients and the doctors treating them, and the emphasis placed on advocacy. Close networks with the voluntary sector are essential and self-care is very important. The rewards are less immediate and visible, but in my experience more intrinsically motivating and lasting.

What makes humanitarian general practice different?

In a climate of austerity, NHS cuts, increasing racism, hate crime and a toxic environment around immigration, being a GP for people seeking asylum is becoming more challenging, but at the same time more important. Forced migration is a phenomenon that is increasing with globalisation. We now have record levels with 65 million people displaced across the world fleeing conflict and human rights violations.

Our challenge is to provide equitable care and fulfil our obligations under the 1951 UN convention. I am not an immigration solicitor. I am not there to decide people's asylum claims, but to provide primary health care to people who have an entitlement to it. In medicine we are trained to believe our patients unless we have clear evidence to the contrary. It is a basic tenet of what we do. Sometimes I am the first person who has listened to a forced migrant without overt judgment or a demand for proof about their history. This therapeutic listening is important for patients. Simple things like saying "I'll do my best to help you" are hugely reassuring to someone who has experienced betrayal and is very far from their usual sources of support. Building a relationship with a person who is mistrustful and feels nobody is on his or her side is satisfying.

I have been able to fine-tune my communication skills through working with interpreters and learning how to write effective letters about medical evidence. Cultural sensibility is a challenge, but the effort to take account of an individual's experience and their interpretation of what it means to them is rewarded with fascinating insights into life, health care and geo-politics from across the globe.

The wider determinants of health and wellbeing often mean that my focus is lower down in Maslow's hierarchy of need. A man with diabetes arriving from Africa in December in flip-flops needs shoes before he needs an HbA1c result to target. A woman who does not know where the next meal is coming from is not interested in her cholesterol level or her Qrisk. My concern becomes nutritional such as iron deficiency anaemia.

There is surprisingly little tropical medicine involved. In 11 years I have not encountered a single case of malaria. One patient had filariasis, but she knew that already so I did not get to make an exciting diagnosis. Problems are similar to the ones we experience here. They may however have been neglected and complications can be more advanced. I think of tuberculosis more quickly as a differential diagnosis than with mainstream patients and, because it is generally a young male population, sexual health is always on my radar.

The bulk of the work involves mental health. It is useful to think in terms of pre-exile, exile and post-exile stressors. All of these contribute to complex psychological trauma. This proves difficult in our traditional models of mental health care. It is hard to have a 'goal orientated to therapy' in PTSD when stress is ongoing and unresolved. People can be hypervigilant and socially isolated. Having no permission to work and consequent loss of status brings challenges to their self-identity. Many talk about not recognising the person they have become and hopelessness is common.

Re-establishing a sense of autonomy and control is difficult with the threat of detention or deportation. I am quicker to medicate first line in an attempt to control symptoms, contradicting NICE guidelines, because of the patients' social and financial contexts. People who do not have adequate support and sometimes little understanding of a western model of psychological health find it hard to engage with therapy. The levels of trauma and perceived lack of progress can also overwhelm the therapists.

Situations where you would usually pick up the phone and ask for help from a statutory body become more perplexing with those who have no recourse to public funds, or limited entitlements. Vulnerable adults and sometimes children are not entitled to the same level of protection afforded to our indigenous population. When alternative solutions are needed my relationships and networks with non-governmental organisations (NGOs) become more important. Some people may say this is not my job as a GP; it is a social work role. But what happens when people do not have rights to care from statutory social work?

It is with dread that I answer the 'what do you do?' question in some social situations. A heavy debate on the rights of migrants is not what I need in my time off. It can be a conversation stopper or leave people feeling flat if you do not handle it carefully. Luckily, I have other outlets for my frustration – mainly riding my bike in all weathers.

Other aspects of the job

I realised early on that just turning up and doing a clinic was never going to be enough to improve the health of people seeking asylum in the United Kingdom. I had no experience of medical politics and no desire to be involved in management, but threatened with cuts that challenged the fundamental principles of 'care according to need' in the NHS, I was compelled to act at different levels and lobby for better provision of care. I have written for international journals, an undertaking I had never imagined doing. The patients' fear of being charged for care has already had an impact on their help-seeking behaviour and I feel it my duty to contest this, discrimination in the NHS and other barriers to their access to health care.

A key principal in this advocacy work has been involvement of refugees themselves in challenging the systems that provide their care. I have facilitated this through linking with agencies in the voluntary sector to avoid any conflicts of interest and breaches of professional boundaries with my own patients. The frustrations come with widespread recognition of need but no political will at higher levels to commission services.

Publicity is a double-edged sword. It is a complex area and unless a sympathetic journalist allows sufficient time to explore it, then comments can be taken out of context. I have turned down media opportunities, such as national TV, when they have only offered a 2-min slot.

Working as a senior clinical lecturer in medical education has given me access to a wide audience of young medics. I am passionate about teaching and regularly deliver sessions on asylum health care for Vocational Training Scheme (VTS) groups and medical student societies. Students have seemed less politically aware in the last decade but that is changing. They understand their agency better and are requesting inclusion of training on helping vulnerable migrants in their curricula. Global Health is becoming trendy but does not require foreign travel anymore – it is on our doorstep in all of our cities.

Self-care is essential to sustainable working in this sector where there is a high risk of vicarious traumatisation. Surrounding yourself with people who support your actions and understand the emotional content of your work is vital because there are lots of knock backs. I have been lucky to have good psychological supervision from Freedom from Torture in the northwest. My GP colleagues at the university and my family all actively support what I do. Rescue cups of tea are vital and this work brings teams closely together. I find you stop 'sweating the small stuff' and all pull together more than in some mainstream primary care teams.

Career options in humanitarian general practice

There are few NHS services commissioned specifically for these roles; however a GP almost everywhere will have migrant patients. Many will be reluctant to disclose their status for fear of being judged or charged for care, but a friendly enquiry and re-affirmation of confidentiality can help you understand their predicament.

Options in the voluntary sector exist in pockets. Organisations such as Freedom from Torture, The Helen Bamber Foundation and Medical Justice offer excellent training for completing Medico-legal reports under the Istanbul Protocol, and visiting detention centres. Doctors of the World UK run Project London, helping unregistered migrants to access mainstream care.

Several medical NGOs have sprung up in response to the recent migrant crisis in Europe. Often the essential roles for medics are not actually delivering hands-on care but raising funds and providing managerial or leadership support from behind the scenes. The larger, better-known NGOs such as Médecins sans Frontières like to recruit GPs. Generalists with the ability to make quick assessments and decisions are very useful in the field. Expert communicators are assets and GPs do not need complicated or expensive equipment. We are great at working in teams. Many projects are based on delivering community health care and a strong interest in public health and delivering education is helpful.

How to become a humanitarian GP

There is no formal or recognised qualification or career path to doing this work. The requirement is grit, determination and having 'a heart' for it. It can be hard, poorly paid, unpredictable and emotionally draining work. You have to actively want to do it. Job security can be an issue with services often precariously funded and contracts short. I have previously been made redundant from an NHS role for asylum seekers, something I never imagined would happen in my career and very damaging at the time for my self-confidence.

Some colleagues like myself are returnees from overseas aid work with organisations such as Médecins sans Frontières and have invaluable practical experience in refugee camps. Their training is superb. Refugee camps can be unhealthy and violent places so the support of an established and respected NGO is crucial for your own safety. I worked in different settings: a TB and kala-azar project in South Sudan; a cholera epidemic on the Thai-Burmese border, a women's health project for internally displaced persons in Afghanistan and a rural health clinic in Liberia. You may have little choice in where you go and flexibility is a key attribute.

Some have studied tropical medicine or international public health. Some have worked for charitable organisations in the United Kingdom such as Project London (Doctors of the World) or faith-based organisations. They have fallen into the roles through demonstrating willing to do locum cover at practices for asylum seekers and refugees, or engaging in this area by seeking out extra training as medical students or GP registrars.

Resources are sparse and even if funding were available for additional training few courses currently exist. Most of us have learned by experience, discussion and sharing ideas through informal networks. Organisations such as WONCA help connect other clinicians from across the world doing similar work.

MY EXPERIENCE

Dr. Rebecca Farrington
University of Manchester

Rose is a chemistry teacher from Africa. She came to us hungry, really hungry, on a Monday morning. She ate my banana, the nurse's sandwich and drank a cup of sweet tea before she was able to talk. Her asylum case was refused and she was too scared of deportation – anticipating a raid on her home by immigration officers at 5 am – to stay in her accommodation. She had taken her children to sleep at the house of 'a man' she knew. Over the weekend she had enough money to feed them beans and toast, but none for herself. 'The man' had given her whisky to drink, to 'make her feel better'. Rose could not disclose what he had asked of her in return for shelter. She said she felt too ashamed.

This consultation was never going to take 10 mins. We first needed to help her feel safe. We needed good quality, independent interpretation and to make sure she understood exactly what confidentiality means. That interpreter needed to deal with her tears, just as we did. We had to reassure her that we were not there to decide her asylum claim, but to provide the health care for which she was entitled. I say 'we' because all of this was a team approach.

We had to assess the risks for Rose's children. I called their head teacher who was fabulous. On weekdays they had free school lunches, but she also made sure they had breakfast. She had checked they were warm and washed, brought them snacks for break time and found them some more second-hand uniforms and shoes when they grew.

Rose felt hopeless. Her options were limited and she was tired of life. She was unable to see a future and had frequent thoughts of suicide. She had decided to push her pram under a lorry and to jump after it. This way at least the older children 'would have a chance' in her thinking. But clearly she was not thinking straight. It was a challenge for us to involve safeguarding and maintain her trust in us.

It quickly became apparent that her experiences before fleeing Africa had a profound impact on Rose's ability to function. The cognitive impairment and re-experiencing symptoms of PTSD had made recall and disclosure of rape and torture too difficult. Re-traumatisation, shame and fear that her children would find out had meant only partial disclosure to the Home Office of what else had happened when her husband was killed in front of her.

As her primary care team we were able to direct her to a female solicitor and provide her with enough medical evidence for the solicitor to commission an independent medicolegal report under the Istanbul protocol. We involved secondary care mental health services, explaining to Rose that she was not 'crazy' as she thought, but unwell. We supported her recovery using continuity of care and our links with a wide range of organisations, statutory and voluntary. We helped keep her family together.

Rose was eventually given temporary refugee status to remain in the United Kingdom for 5 years. The relief on her face at finally being able to look after her children in safety was reward enough for our team.

Conclusions

The Inverse Care Law is alive and well more than 40 years on from Julian Tudor Hart's original article.[1] Forced migrants are amongst the most vulnerable people in our communities, yet many lack access to primary health care in a way that is meaningful. Being a GP for this group is about more than ploughing your way through surgery. It can be shocking and frustrating, but it also gives you an insight to the wider world and a chance to meet people who have survived experiences beyond your imagination. It requires patience and determination. Helping them become healthy and thrive against the odds is a slow process, but it can be immensely fulfilling.

'Altruism' seems insufficient to describe my motivation for this work. That feels very one sided. During the past 11 years I have met and learned from some incredible people. Many who have stood up for their beliefs and then suffered the consequences. I am in awe of them and consider it a privilege to be part of their journeys.

THE ACADEMIC GP

PROFESSOR ALISTAIR HAY

Centre for Academic Primary Care, University of Bristol

Academic GPs are essential to our discipline. Our role is to inspire, teach, inform and improve the lives of our patients and colleagues through the acquisition of new generalisable knowledge – research.

Change is a constant feature of health care provision internationally, and university centres of academic primary care (often led by GP professors) provide the teaching to prepare the next generation of GPs, and the research evidence to ensure changes are safe, effective and a sensible use of resource.

We work in highly professionalised, multidisciplinary teams to answer questions, such as 'Are primary care nurse led clinics as clinically effective as doctor led clinics and which is most cost effective?'; 'Is primary care providing more appointments today compared with 10 years ago?'; and 'Should corticosteroids be used for adults presenting to primary care with Bell's palsy?'.

Although academia fits the personalities of some GPs, and may therefore help prevent burnout, the multiple competing demands require careful management.

What makes academic general practice different?

For me, academic general practice is first and foremost about the application of ideas to practice. To develop novel thinking requires imagination – to see beyond today's practice, and ask 'what if ...' or 'how could we ...' questions. For example, a question that has preoccupied me for 20 years is how could we improve the use of antibiotics in primary care. The ideas come from reading around a subject, hearing what others are considering, from within and outside our discipline, and considering how these might improve practice.

Once the general idea is clear, it is converted into an aim, usually with subsidiary objectives. This could be a teaching aim (e.g. 'to improve medical students' knowledge, skills and attitudes regarding strategies to improve the use of antibiotics in health care') or a research question (e.g. 'Are corticosteroids clinically effective in reducing the unwanted symptoms of lower respiratory tract infections in adults presenting to primary care?').

Once the aim and objectives are clear, the optimal method to achieve the aim is selected. And this is where training in teaching and research methods is needed – so the academic is aware of the 'tools in the toolkit'. For example, there is strong evidence that enhanced communication skills safely reduce antibiotic prescribing.[2] For a second-year medical student unfamiliar with how to consult and intimidated by talking to patients, the rudimentaries of this high-level skill are probably best acquired through observed practice with simulated patients. If a randomised controlled trial is to be conducted to establish the effectiveness of corticosteroids for acute lower respiratory tract infection, a necessary first step is to summarise existing evidence, usually by conducting a systematic review.[3]

In contrast to clinical practice (where we are largely in 'reactive' mode), academic time is largely spent being 'proactive'. If you do not take the initiative it will not happen.

As far as patients are concerned, although you will have less time in your practice than most GPs, the academic GP should be largely indistinguishable from their non-academic colleagues. By taking ownership of patients' problems, it is possible to provide continuity of care, and the fewer days spent in practice allow us to bring more energy when we are present. Personally, I have always resisted the temptation to call myself 'professor' in my practice, mainly out of respect for my non-academic colleagues, whom I regard as more qualified and clinically expert, but also to avoid seeing all the most difficult patients!

So, how does an academic spend his or her time when not at the practice? The simple answer is 'it depends'. The more complex answer is that 'no 2 weeks are the same' and that non-clinical time is hugely varied. Many GP academics enjoy high levels of autonomy and choice over the balance of time between teaching, research, university and non-university work (such as sitting on national committees).

To progress, all academics must meet the metrics of success stipulated by the university sector, which is a highly competitive environment. Most universities prize grant income and published papers ('publish or perish') above all else, while also requiring active engagement in teaching and the demonstration that research is making a difference in the real world (so-called 'impact'). Research grants are awarded competitively with between 10% and 25% of all grants funded. Papers reporting research have to meet with the approval of peers (peer review) before journals will publish.

Other aspects of the job

While informing patient care through teaching and research, most of the role does not involve direct, face-to-face care. GP partners are responsible for running the business of their practice, with increasing academic seniority, so the managerial responsibilities of leading research groups grow. With a small group, they are responsible for deciding the research questions the group will address, along with hiring and managing group members. More senior academic GPs are responsible for setting the strategic direction and culture of their centres and many go on to senior leadership positions within the university structures. This might include becoming the dean of a faculty or medical school, where they are responsible for teaching curricula and the research priorities of institutes.

There are also opportunities outside of the university structure. Many academic GPs sit on (and chair) NICE guideline development groups, government advisory groups and national grant funding bodies. There are other national organisations requiring leadership and administration, such as the RCGP and the Society for Academic Primary Care.

Working with industry affords the opportunity to increase the 'real-world' impact of research. An example would be working with software companies to develop apps for clinical care or point of care diagnostic devices.

Career options in academic general practice

The career options for the academic GP are endless and are largely determined by the interests and commitment of the academic. The process can be likened to the differentiation of stem cells. The early academic (rather like the medical student) has the potential to become almost any senior academic (type of doctor). How you 'differentiate' is largely up to you and your interests.

That said, there are tough choices to be made. Many universities (but not all) expect academic GPs to see patients, teach, do research and administer elements of university life. In my opinion, it is possible to do two of these to a very high standard – and one must be clinical care. This means most academics have to choose between majoring on research or teaching.

Those who prioritise teaching will be responsible for how the requirements of the General Medical Council's vision for the training of doctors are delivered. Primary care has an excellent reputation for delivering high-quality teaching, such that many medical schools are increasing the amount of teaching delivered in primary care. Many academic GPs also conduct pedagogical research to determine optimal teaching methods.

If you major on research, then most academic GPs develop a specialist area of interest in which they acquire expertise and reputation. You are likely to have considerable choice over the topic, though your early decisions are likely to be influenced by the senior academics around you. And thanks to the National Institute for Health Research (NIHR), there has never been a better time to start a research active academic career in general practice. Set up by Professor Dame Sally Davies in 2006, the NIHR's raison d'être is to conduct research for patient benefit. Its priorities are close to those of primary care research putting us in a strong position to secure grant funding.

How to become an academic GP

Becoming a senior academic GP will take many years of dedicated study and commitment, while maintaining your abilities as a clinician. You will have MRCGP (and often other medical qualifications such as MRCP, DCH, DRCOG) and a higher research degree (PhD/MD) often now preceded by a Masters (MSc) in primary care, public health or research methods. But what of the attributes of a successful academic GP? In my opinion, they need to:

- Be curious, enjoying reading around ideas and following them through to their logical conclusions
- Be able to assimilate existing, and generate new, ideas
- Enjoy problem solving

- Cope with (better still enjoy) being at the centre of rapid developments and changes
- Be able to think clearly and specify project aims, objectives and methods
- Be excellent communicators – able to convey ideas in writing and verbally
- Be able to enthuse and inspire – medical students, members of research groups and committees
- Be willing to support and mentor careers
- Be able to lead, teach and facilitate large groups (lectures) and small groups and 1-2-1 (e.g. PhD students) and be able to adapt quickly to changing group dynamics and 'curve balls' from students
- Be committed to using research and teaching to improve the discipline of general practice
- There is now a clear, highly professionalised (albeit highly competitive), academic career structure, which might take the following steps:
  - Complete MB ChB (or equivalent), taking all opportunities to interact with academic GPs, such as student selected components and intercalated BSc.
  - Academic F2 – this will be your first taste of academia and allows you to work on a teaching or research project under the supervision of a senior, experienced academic.
  - Clinical Academic Fellow. This is your first serious step into academia, allowing you to add a 4 year to your standard 3 years as a Specialist Trainee in general practice. Instead of completing your final 12 months full-time in general practice, you do 50:50 clinical: academic for 2 years, again under the supervision of a senior, experienced academic. Here you start to gain your teaching and research skills, often completing an MSc. If you know what you want to teach or research, then you may deliberately seek to work in a centre with a strong reputation in that area. Towards the end of this period, you will be starting to think about applying for funding to do a PhD.
  - Doctoral fellow, usually externally funded through competitive application to the NIHR or the Medical Research Council. This is where you gain your true research colours. A PhD is a serious undertaking (minimum of 3 years' full-time equivalent) during which you develop expertise in research methods and a research topic and produce novel research of publishable quality.
  - With your PhD you can then apply for a postdoctoral research fellow or university lecturer position. If following a research pathway, you will continue to develop the ideas started in your PhD, still with some supervision, but while developing the skills to become an independent researcher.
  - A Senior Lecturer will be starting to secure modest grant funding as Principal Investigator (the independent research leader). You will be developing the skills to lead small- to medium-sized projects, working with experts from other disciplines, such as statisticians, health economists and sociologists. You will be developing a national reputation for

your work, resulting in invitations to speak at national meetings and conferences.

- A Reader is usually 'on track' to become a professor and by this time in his or her career, the academic is leading large, multicentre, internationally competitive grants and leading significant elements of university life, such as teaching units or being responsible for the training programmes of PhD students. You will have a growing international reputation for your work, resulting in invitations to speak at international conferences and meetings.

MY EXPERIENCE

Professor Alistair Hay
University of Bristol

After completing GP training in 2007 my first taster as an academic was at the University of Leicester (1997–2001) where I was fortunate to secure a position to allow me to complete a MD (medical equivalent PhD) while practising 50:50 as an associate GP.

I then secured a lectureship at the University of Bristol in 2001 where I have remained to date, becoming a professor in 2013. It was only latterly that I felt I moved from being a 'GP trying to be an academic', to an 'academic trying to be a GP'.

A large part of my academic life has been lived during the lifetime of the NIHR. This has promoted 'applied research for patient benefit', very much playing to the types of research that academic GPs conduct, and allowed me to be highly research active and secure several research fellowships, culminating in a NIHR Research Professorship.

In the past 10 years I have worked with highly talented individuals from a broad range of academic disciplines based at the universities of Bristol, Cardiff, London, Nottingham, Oxford and Southampton.

In addition to supporting others' leadership of research, I have chaired a NICE guideline[4] and led studies to improve the use of antibiotics in primary care.

Conclusions

Life as an academic GP is never dull – you will have a huge variety of responsibilities and autonomy. You have considerable flexibility and freedom to manage your time as you see fit and the pleasure of working with other bright, interested and interesting academics committed to improving primary care. You will also enjoy opportunities to travel and learn first-hand how other countries address the challenges of delivering, researching and teaching general practice.

Whether it is a recipe for, or a strategy to prevent, burnout will depend on the individual, but it is not something to be done lightly and you must enjoy its upsides to endure its inevitable challenges. Although you will have more flexibility to work around other commitments, there are few academics I know who do not work at least some evenings, weekends and holidays.

For me, the main excitement lies in the development of new, preferably elegant, ideas which generate novel evidence to inform the clinical practice of the future and ultimately improve the lives of our patients and colleagues.

THE EDUCATIONAL GP

DR. EUAN LAWSON

Director of Community Studies, Faculty of Health, and Medicine, Lancaster University

'In seeking wisdom, the first step is silence, the second listening, the third remembering, the fourth practicing, the fifth -- teaching others.'

Solomon ibn Gabirol
11th Century poet and philosopher

There are many different ways to get involved with medical education. Broadly, these can be split into undergraduate and postgraduate opportunities. In each of these there is a range of different career options. It is possible to work full-time in medical education, and yet it is one of the best areas to incorporate into a portfolio career with a multitude of different posts and sessional work being the norm.

What makes medical education different?

One of the things that makes medical education special is that shared experience; we have all been through the process. There are no health care professionals who have not themselves been learners and, of course, we are all lifelong learners in the context of continuing to maintain our professional skills and knowledge. Teaching is a natural progression for many health care professionals as they move through their careers. It is also an expected part of the profession with the GMC explicitly stating in Good Medical Practice that doctors should be prepared to contribute to teaching and training.[5]

As one delves further into this speciality it soon becomes apparent that there is a whole host of potential niches to explore and develop. It may be academic medical education and research, it may be related to managing learners in difficulty, it could be developing simulation for surgical trainees, or promoting resilience in undergraduates. There are many different options that fall under the umbrella of medical education.

Almost anyone can stand up and be a medical educator insofar as they can deliver a lecture. We have all been to lectures where the thought given to this deceptively simple process has not extended beyond the most rudimentary of principles. We have all been subjected to some appalling learning experiences as we have developed as undergraduates and once qualified. Many lecturers are inspiring but modern medical education is now rarely about the delivery of lectures.

Other aspects of the job

As well as teaching in various formats, undergraduate tutors can expect to be involved in a full range of responsibilities in their medical school. For example, your main role may be teaching small groups of medical students clinical knowledge around a specific topic. However, it is likely you will also need to be involved in activities such as writing exam questions, designing and delivering an objective structured clinical examination (OSCE), taking students under your wing as a mentor, liaising with local GP and community placements, designing and implementing quality assurance processes for teaching, peer reviewing colleagues and so on. This is all in addition to the basic requirements to develop and deliver high-quality learning materials that work for a full range of students, no matter what their learning styles and takes into account the variations in baseline knowledge.

Career options in medical education

Many of these posts offer flexible timings that can be fitted in and around existing clinical work and other responsibilities with some pre-planning. The flexibility makes it particularly helpful in terms of incorporating medical education into one's career. It is perfectly possible, and indeed is probably the route followed by most people, where a strand of work is developed further over time. Most people will start with a few sessions and this may then blossom into a special interest over time.

Of course, there is no necessity to develop a full-time career in medical education. It is a career option that can be easily blended into clinical practice or other responsibilities. Most medical educators find time spent with learners invigorating and this feeds back into quality care in their clinical work. The opportunity to take a step back from clinical work, to reflect on it in the context of delivering teaching is particularly valuable and is likely to make a considerable difference in sustaining a long-term career and avoiding burnout.

How to get involved in medical education

UNDERGRADUATES OPPORTUNITIES

Almost all medical schools will employee GPs and doctors in various capacities to contribute to their teaching as part of their curricula. Typical opportunities might involve facilitating problem-based learning groups, teaching communication skills and teaching small group tutorials clinical topics across the full range of primary care specialities. In addition, there may be a requirement for delivering lectures or plenaries, and this is more likely to be the case if you have a particular niche within which you are a GP specialist.

There may also be opportunities to convene special study or elective modules depending on the exact structure of the curriculum at your local medical school. These can provide valuable experience and are highly flexible.

POSTGRADUATE OPPORTUNITIES

There are many postgraduate opportunities in the field of medical education. These are more variable than undergraduate opportunities and will be largely dependent on the organisations and the topics from which you choose to get involved. You may be involved in delivering education sessions around specific specialist knowledge that you have.

GP tutors are often involved across the country in providing local postgraduate education opportunities. There are also numerous private companies who provide educational materials for GPs, and you may be involved in writing and developing online articles, journal articles or e-modules. All of these need to be designed in accordance with good principles of curriculum development, delivered in an effective way that works for a range of learners and quality assured to ensure the materials can evolve and be responsive to learners' needs.

GP tutors may also be involved in managing doctors or other health care professionals who are in difficulty for various reasons. Some of this work may overlap with that of GP appraisers.

LEARNERS IN PRACTICE

One obvious way to develop involvement in medical education is to get involved as a GP trainer. This will suit GPs who are well established and settled in practice. The process of becoming a trainer will typically require that you hold MRCGP and have been on the National Performers' List for a minimum of 3 years. Each region runs Trainers' Course that covers the principles of being an educator in primary care. Some of these will be linked to formal qualifications such as a Postgraduate Certificate in Medical Education.

For those who do not wish the long-term commitment of becoming a GP trainer, then the option of hosting undergraduate students may work well. Currently, around 42% of practices across the United Kingdom take medical students, and it is very likely your local medical school will have placements to fill.[6] Training is offered and commitments can be flexible to fit with existing practice circumstances. Educational opportunities to train practice nurses, physician associates and Foundation Year doctors may also be available.

WORKING AS AN APPRAISER

Working as an appraiser falls under the remit of medical education as a formative developmental process. There are some who would argue that this has been tested in recent years as appraisal has morphed into revalidation. This will depend on your underlying philosophy and perspective towards the appraisal process. If you regard appraisal as a formative developmental process that is there to enhance and support lifelong learning, then there is a clear link to medical education. However, the cogs of revalidation are also continuing to turn, and there are some mandatory requirements which not all medical educators will necessarily feel comfortable when they fall within their remit as appraisers.

However, undoubtedly appraisals are often regarded by appraisers as a positive experience where they get to network and support colleagues. They are tremendously flexible with appraisers and can fit easily into just about any working pattern. The time and date of the appraisal is mutually agreed, and the appraiser then has to find the time to review materials before the meetings and complete the documentation. There will be mandatory developmental sessions for appraisers, but these tend not to be burdensome once the initial training has been completed.

How to become an educational GP

Perhaps the most important quality to be a medical educator is enthusiasm. It is strongly recommended you have a least a modicum of it before getting involved with medical education. The communication skills we cherish as GPs all come into play to manage relationships with learners and to handle sensitively the process of helping to guide learners through their careers.

There are several postgraduate medical education qualifications available across the country. It is well worth considering these at an early point in your career. A Postgraduate Certificate in Medical Education provides a solid foundation in the principles of teaching, curriculum design and assessment. They will provide an important grounding in the most important aspects of medical education in which ever area you specialise in. Topics such as curriculum design, feedback, assessment and standard-setting, the role of simulation and other areas are all put in their appropriate academic context. The underlying literature of medical education shares more with the social sciences than the more familiar biomedical literature. This in itself is a valuable developmental strand that can open up new vistas to doctors brought up on with a philosophical approach that owes more to positivism.

Some medical education roles can be quite competitive, and a postgraduate qualification will also give an edge in any applications. In addition, most students find it personally satisfying and it significantly enhances and improves their own experience and engagement with learners in all areas. There are distance learning options available as well as other programs which adopt a more blended learning approach, sitting alongside more traditional face-to-face programs. Overall, there is almost certainly a postgraduate program that will work for you.

MY EXPERIENCE

Dr. Euan Lawson
Lancaster University

In 2006 I left my salaried GP post and started to locum regularly in the North Lancashire and South Lakes area. I was put in contact with the new medical school at Lancaster University, and I worked on a sessional basis delivering communication skills sessions to Y1 medical students. At the start this was for one session every couple of weeks and I also worked as a PBL facilitator for 3 sessions every 2 weeks during term time. Over the coming months and years, I delivered the occasional lecture and helped out with any clinical teaching that was needed. Around this time I also applied for and took up a post, Community Clinical Tutor, for 1 day per week teaching Y4 Liverpool medical students in Barrow-in-Furness. So, I quickly built up a portfolio of 1–2 days of medical education roles over the course of the next year or two. I worked as a locum when I did not have teaching responsibilities. I also helped out with local OSCEs and looked for other opportunities to get involved in medical education.

In the following years, I took on a role as a GP appraiser and this culminated in involvement as GP Appraisal Lead for Cumbria. The role with Lancaster Medical School also grew. In addition, I was involved in a project to deliver postgraduate education to GPs on the topic of hepatitis B and C – an offshoot of my clinical interest in substance misuse management. I have also been involved in accrediting education events for the RCGP and writing educational materials for e-modules and professional resources such as patient.info.

All of these activities have been paid and most of have been very flexible. I have been able to build my own working pattern – one that is sustainable and reduces the risk of burnout. One of the most useful things I did early in my involvement in medical education was to complete a PGCert Med Ed. This gave me a theoretical understanding of medical education that underpinned the more practical aspects of the job.

At any point in my involvement in medical education, I could have settled on that level of involvement. I have never been under pressure to do more and I have been able to enjoy a diverse portfolio career for the past 10 years. I have been involved with Lancaster Medical School since its start and, clearly, that is an unusual event. However, there are opportunities across the country. Building medical education into one's career is a great option to provide a refreshing change from the daily clinical grind. It also feeds back into that clinical work and creates a virtuous circle.

Conclusions

Overall, medical education offers a multitude of opportunities for enthusiastic GPs to engage with learners at a formative stage of their careers as well as with established health care professionals. There is a wide range of possible levels of involvement and it is a rewarding dimension to add to your career. In addition, it can be seamlessly blended with a clinical interest that will go a long way to ensuring your career is sustainable and stimulating.

"The mediocre teacher tells. The good teacher explains. The superior teacher demonstrates. The great teacher inspires."

William Arthur Ward

Resource

The Academy of Medical Educators (www.medicaleducators.org) was formed in 2006 with the aim of the advancement of medical education for public benefit. They offer the opportunity to apply for membership or fellowship depending on your current experience. Applications for these are based on a portfolio approach that will fit well with annual appraisal requirements.

REFERENCES

1. Tudor Hart J. The inverse care law. *Lancet* 1971;297(7696):405–12.
2. Little P, Stuart B, Francis N, Douglas E, Tonkin-Crine S, Anthierens S, Cals JW, et al. Effects of internet-based training on antibiotic prescribing rates for acute respiratory-tract infections: A multinational, cluster, randomised, factorial, controlled trial. *Lancet* 2013;382(9899):1175–82.
3. El-Gohary M, Hay AD, Coventry P, Moore M, Stuart B, Little P. Corticosteroids for acute and subacute cough following respiratory tract infection: A systematic review. *Fam Pract* 2013;30(5):9.
4. NICE. *Antimicrobial stewardship: systems and processes for effective antimicrobial medicine use*, National Institute for Health and Care Excellence: London. 2015.
5. GMC. *Good medical practice.* General Medical Council; 2013. http://www.gmc-uk.org/guidance/good_medical_practice.asp (accessed 3 April 2017).
6. Derbyshire H, Rees E, Gay SP, McKinley RK. Undergraduate teaching in UK general practice: A geographical snapshot. *Br J Gen Pract* 2014;64(623):e336–45.

7

Resilience

DR. EUAN LAWSON
Director of Community Studies, Faculty of Health and
Medicine, Lancaster University

The first questions that anyone might ask about resilience are: 'What is it? How do I know whether I have resilience? And, how do I develop it? There are few easy answers to these questions, but there is an emerging consensus on some of the factors involved.

When the term 'resilience' is applied to materials, it refers to a quality that allows for it to be bent, stretched or compressed and still return to its original shape. It is easy to think of this as a metaphor for resilience in people. It is the ability to bounce back from adversity.

Lown et al. define resilience as follows, and this closely fits with a similar definition from the American Psychological Association: 'There are many definitions of resilience but it is best considered as the individual's ability to adapt to and manage stress and adversity: essential qualities for GPs'.[1]

Southwick and Charney have studied the quality of resilience in people who have been through trauma, both physical and psychological. Some had experienced trauma through being a soldier in a warzone, or through being the victim of a terrorist attack. Others had experienced trauma due to physical and sexual assaults, or perhaps through being involved in serious road traffic collisions. They noted that resilence is 'complex, multidimensional and dynamic in nature'.[2]

Resilience is not a fixed commodity. It can vary across the life course, it could vary from month to month even, and it can also vary depending on the exact nature of the stressor. There are various tests that can measure resilience, and these tests are generally self-reported using Likert scales. They are most useful for research and are less helpful for aiding the creation of day-to-day strategies for individuals.

NEUROBIOLOGY OF RESILIENCE

This is worth dwelling on. One might assume resilience is a rather wishy-washy new age term that is nebulous, related to aspects of personality or other inner qualities that are undefinable. Increasingly, neuroscience is mapping out the specific pathways where resilience is found, and this leads to credible strategies to address concerns when those pathways bend or break.

Acute stress response

This is how the mind and the body respond to persistent stress. We all know the hormones that rise in these circumstances: the fight-or-flight surge of adrenaline and catecholamines. There is a rise in cortisol levels and also in pro-inflammatory cytokines. These are primitive responses, enormously helpful in the course of evolution to preserve us from short-term hazards. In modern life, these responses do not necessarily ebb away, and this persistent stress activation can damage us with changes in the brain tissue and maladaption in the hypothalamic-pituitary-adrenal axis. This persistent stress is associated with chronic illnesses including cardiovascular disease.

The problem with sustained stress is that it impairs decision making. Martin et al. highlight other impacts[3]:

- Interference with empathy and communication
- Narrowing of the field of vision (literally and metaphorically)
- Decrease in generosity
- Decrease in cooperativeness
- Increase in xenophobia
- Increased likelihood if interpreting ambiguous expressions as hostile
- Increased likelihood of displacing frustration and aggression onto those around us

As David Peters puts it, 'it makes us more dull-witted and less friendly'.[4] As these responses kick in, it has been shown that compassion and empathy diminish. Clearly, this is not ideal for anybody, and it is particularly worrying in the medical profession. However, this is a feature of medical training in general. There tends to be a decline in empathy over the course of training with an increase in 'professional numbing'.

PHYSICIAN PERSONALITY AND RESILIENCE

Physician personality has been found to be associated with wellness. One Norwegian study found that neuroticism and conscientiousness traits predict stress in medical students.[5] Workaholism and perfectionism have been traits associated with suicide in physicians.[6] Lemaire and Wallace explored personality and doctors' perceptions with a cross-sectional study that surveyed more than

1000 Canadian physicians.[7] They had previously noted that physicians tended to identify strongly (%) with three different personality types (Figure 7.1):

- Workaholic personality – 53%
- Type A personality – 62%
- Control freak personality – 36%

They also compared the physicians who identified with these personalities with those who did not. Specifically, they wanted to see how they differed in how they perceived the impact of personality on professional performance and how they experienced wellness.

They found that most of the physicians did identify with at least one of these personalities. The workaholic personality was associated with one potentially harmful and three positive wellbeing outcomes. The control freak personality was associated with five potentially harmful outcomes.

There are several factors in play with physician personalities. There is an issue with selection, but there is also a culture within medicine that can exacerbate existing traits in physicians. Personalities themselves may not be malleable, but awareness amongst physicians of their own potential vulnerabilities, their inherent resilience and their ability to withstand burnout is crucial to manage clinician wellness.

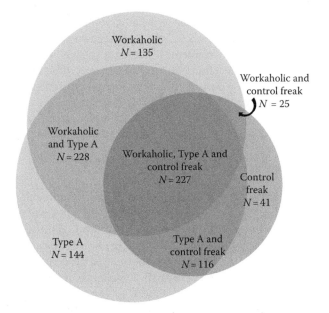

Figure 7.1 Proportions of 916 Respondents Who Identified with One, Two or All Three of the Predetermined Personalities. (From Lemaire, J.B., and Wallace, J.E., *BMC Health Serv Res.*, 14, 616, 2014.)

OTHER FEATURES ASSOCIATED WITH RESILIENCE

Charney and Southwick found 10 factors associated with resilience.[2]
Psychological and social factors associated with resilience

- Facing fear: an adaptive response
- Having a moral compass
- Religion and spirituality
- Social support
- Having good role models
- Being physically fit
- Brain fitness: making sure your brain is challenged
- Having 'cognitive and emotional flexibility'
- Having 'meaning, purpose and growth' in life
- 'Realistic' optimism

These are more encouraging because they are not all necessarily fixed traits. They can, potentially, be addressed.

'Realistic' optimism

What do we mean by optimism? Southwick and Charney regard this as a 'future orientated attitude.' Optimists tend to believe that the future will be bright and that good things will happen to people who work hard. Psychologists have developed tests to measure optimism. Some of the most resilient people that have been studied have been the most optimistic. Psychologists have investigated why optimists seem to be particularly resilient. It has been suggested that this leads us back to the fight-or-flight reaction that has already been described. It has been shown that when we have positive emotions it tends to reduce physiological arousal, so there is a direct mechanism to ensure that people get various benefits from their optimism. These are things such as improved attention and ability to actively problem solve as well as our greater interest in socialising.

Facing fear: An adaptive response

This factor associated with resilience is also linked to the fight-or-flight response. Pavlov's dogs and the phenomenon of classical conditioning are familiar to most people. We experience a response such as fear when exposed to a stimulus which would not otherwise cause distress but has been previously associated with some kind of traumatic event. This resilience-associated factor is particularly important to people who have had a very traumatic experience in the past.

Ethics and altruism: Having a moral compass

The reason that Southwick and Charney included this ethics and altruism was because when they interviewed people who had been through trauma, they found that many of the individuals who seem to be particularly resilient had a sense of right and wrong that was particularly valuable to them during periods of extreme stress. They also found that altruism, a concern for the welfare of others, was often part of that value system. Some trauma survivors, particularly those who had been involved in torture, had been forced to face some deeply difficult moral choices. To some extent, this may be less relevant to the medical profession where there is often already a strong code of moral and ethical behaviour. However, there could certainly be value in deepening the links and engagement with that moral compass – working with colleagues who reinforce those ethical positions and sense of altruism could be of particular benefit to health care professionals.

Religion and spirituality

Many people find that their religious beliefs offer them resilience. Southwick and Charney felt this to be as applicable to people who are atheists as to those with strongly held beliefs in any of the world's major religions. The important thing about this factor is that that does not necessarily denote having to believe in a particular God. It is more about people who are comfortable with their place in the universe. That said, many of the most highly resilient individuals were found by Southwick and Charney to have had particularly strong benefits from their spirituality or religion.

Social support

Humans are basically social creatures. Having a social support network has been clearly associated with resilience. It has been shown that social support can promote physical and mental health. And the relationship seems to work both ways – it may even be the case that giving social support is more beneficial for physical health than receiving it. There is an underlying biology of relationships and specific neurobiological changes that occur in the context of relationships have been noted by neuroscientists. In particular, the hormone oxytocin seems to play a strong role in social communication and the formation of a sense of affiliation, as well as in other interactions such as sexual behaviour.

General practice may seem like a highly social activity, but it is entirely possible for general practitioners (GPs) to become very isolated. The work of seeing patients does, by necessity, happen in isolation and behind closed doors. Those interactions with people are not necessarily social in the sense that is beneficial to the GP. GPs may go prolonged periods without the opportunity to socialise with colleagues in a way that promotes their own health.

Wallace and Lemaire studied positive and negative factors associated with physician wellbeing and noted the importance of co-worker support. Interestingly, this study also highlighted the role of patients in wellbeing. While being a source of stress, patients were also an important source of satisfaction and therefore wellbeing for doctors.[8]

Having good role models

In some of the first studies to look at resilience it was shown that the most resilient children usually had at least one person who gave them genuine support and served as a role model. Southwick and Charney found similar findings in their own research. Their research established that everybody needs appropriate, resilient role models. Mentors form the critical role in inspiring and motivating their charges and fostering resilience. How does it work? This seems to be down to imitation – an innate ability and one that we have from the earliest infancy but that persists throughout our lives. Role modelling has been well established in medical education and for trainees at all levels but, perhaps, there could be further development of this area for more senior clinicians.

Being physically fit

The obvious benefits of physical exercise to our physical health seem also to extend to benefits to mental health including improvements to mood and cognition. Most importantly, there seems to be benefit in terms of resilience. There are clear neurobiological mechanisms that explain how this could function. The chemicals that improve mood such as endorphins, serotonin and dopamine are all increased after exercise. In addition the pathways that release cortisol are dampened by exercise. There are other potential mechanisms including neurogenesis which involve the making of new brain cells when specific genes are switched on.

One of the key points to remember about exercise and resilience is that we only get stronger and more physically fit by ensuring we have appropriate rest periods. This is often neglected. Physical exercise itself is the stressor but the adaptation only comes afterward. This means diet and sleep are key factors in developing resilience due to physical activity.

Brain fitness: Making sure your brain is challenged

Southwick and Charney found that people who are lifelong learners tend to have higher levels of resilience. They found that it is possible to do various different activities that can promote both cognitive and emotional improvements in brain function – mental training. There is still some scepticism around 'brain training', but there is certainly good evidence that there is an enormous amount of plasticity inherent in the brain and that this neuroplasticity can be developed in some form. It is also known that the use of techniques such as mindfulness can help us learn how to develop calm and an improved awareness of our emotions and perceptions. Even if people remain sceptical about interventions such as mindfulness, there is clear evidence for cognitive behavioural therapy, an obvious form of mental and emotional training.

Having cognitive and emotional flexibility

Cognitive flexibility is an important factor in resilience. We need to have the ability to accept the reality of the situations that we are in. It is obvious that avoidance and denial are not helpful in coping with changing circumstances. This concept of 'acceptance' has been identified by psychologists as an important ingredient in people being able to tolerate highly stressful circumstances. It has also been shown to be associated with better psychological and physical health.

This is been described by Southwick and Charney as cognitive reappraisal. This cognitive reappraisal can come in many different forms. One potential area is in the shape of gratitude. Resilient people that have been through particularly traumatic events often then appreciate the things they still have. They also suggest that humour is a form of cognitive reappraisal. It is a mechanism to help people reframe events and to face their fears. There is the possibility that it can be used as an avoidance tactic, but for many people the ability to see humour, even in the most tragic of circumstances, is an important factor in resilience.

Having 'meaning, purpose and growth' in life

The 10th factor described by Southwick and Charney is about having a purpose. Those people who have a clear sense of mission often have a very deep resilience and ability to withstand enormous stresses and strains. In many ways, in the United Kingdom, the National Health Service (NHS) has provided many clinicians with that sense of purpose in their clinical practice. As Nigel Lawson, a Conservative politician said, the NHS is 'the closest thing the English have to a religion'. It gives many workers in the NHS a meaning that goes beyond the monthly pay packet. This requirement for meaning and purpose has been shown repeatedly in studies with soldiers who have embarked on missions. However, it has also been of importance in civilian workers who have been able to cope with work-related stress. This factor also highlights a potential unintended consequence of re-organisations and stress within the NHS system; it will, indirectly, erode the resilience of the workers within it.

THE PARADOX

One of the biggest challenges facing the medical profession is the fundamental paradox at the heart of managing burnout. There is an expectation that doctors will be cool, calm, and collected. Confident and yet still caring and empathetic.

These may not be obviously mutually exclusive: the neurobiology of the human brain rather suggests that, to some extent, they are exactly that. Doctors are faced with people going through tremendously intense emotional experiences while unwell. Yet, clinicians need to suppress the parts of the brain – limbic and reptilian – that regard these experiences as highlighting a threat. Patients push our limbic brain buttons, even if it is happening subconsciously.

CLINICAL SUPERVISION

Dr. Rebecca Farrington

GPwSI in Refugee Health, Clinical Lecturer, University of Manchester

Dr. Jude Boyles

Psychological Therapist, Manager of Freedom from Torture
North West Centre in Manchester

As part of my role as a GP for asylum seekers, I sought clinical supervision from Freedom from Torture, a credible and reputable organisation working with a similar group of patients. This has proven essential for me in avoiding vicarious trauma and keeping my work life sustainable. My experiences have helped me realise that clinical supervision is also valuable for GPs in mainstream practice. We are all exposed to extremes of emotion and the difficult lives of our patients on a regular basis. Maintaining our humanity and retaining our compassion are important.

The role of supervision is to provide a reflective space to explore our work with patients: the treatments offered or the relationships and dynamics in the consultation. Sometimes, we find ourselves being confused about our emotional responses to a patient or feel ill equipped to manage a particular presentation. It is not therapy but supervision that gives us a non-judgemental opportunity to examine new or different ways of practicing or communicating. It is a chance to think about the impact of the work and ensure we continue to practice safely, healthily and ethically.

The supervisor should not in any way be personally connected to the supervisee so that they can be as objective as possible. The supervision is confidential, but the supervisor has similar duties to other health care staff in that if the supervisor considers that the practitioner is unsafe to practice or has not acted appropriately around safeguarding, the supervisor is expected to act upon these concerns.

I have found it useful to have a non-GP clinician as my supervisor on a one-to-one basis. Others may find that sharing experiences collectively, such as in Balint groups or Schwarz rounds, suits them better.

Resilience is our ability to soak up that neurobiological stress and not develop the adverse consequences of persistent stress and arousal. The need to develop resilience in trainees has been recognised. In one study GP trainees on a scheme in the south of England were found to have significant levels of burnout in their first year of training.[9] It was also noted that less than half of the trainees were under-estimating their levels of burnout.

If the innate resilience of doctors is being stretched as this early stage in their careers, it suggests that we need to start building on that innate resilience at medical school, during training, and on through our careers, to future proof ourselves against the increasing stresses of our working lives.

GP WELLBEING: LESSONS LEARNED FROM A TRAINEE-LED INITIATIVE

DR. DUNCAN SHREWSBURY
GP Registrar, Chair RCGP AiT Committee

It is unfortunately the case that those training and working within the medical profession are at significantly greater risk of mental illness and suicide than the general public.[10] At a time when junior doctor morale in the United Kingdom was believed to be at a nadir, several cases where junior doctors had turned to suicide were reported in the UK mainstream media.[11] This highlighted the issue of morale, but also wellbeing. Anecdotally, trainees experienced a lack of understanding, empathy or even basic kindness when approaching colleagues and seniors for support with issues relating to distress caused by their own mental illness, or that of peers.

GP trainees on the Royal College of General Practitioners (RCGP) Associates in Training committee wanted to take action to address this issue. We collectively felt saddened, disappointed and incensed that a colleague or friend would find himself or herself in a situation where the only option that they felt able to take was to end their own life. Even more, we felt that the rhetoric around such tragedies, and the response that trainees received to similar problems, denied the sympathy and humanity that we would wish to afford our own patients in times of great distress.

At a February meeting of the whole committee, we discussed and developed an idea to address the situation. We wanted to support a vision of happy, healthy colleagues who were able to invest in and maintain their wellbeing. We wanted to change the conversation around needing, seeking and providing help for doctors experiencing difficulty. However, we acknowledged the challenge of stigma around such issues and were wary of adding to negativity. The simple idea of trying to achieve change positively prompted us to look wider. We drew on ideas from positive psychology (literally, the study of how positive outcomes are achieved,[12] rather than the study of pathological psychology), and took inspiration from work done in the teaching profession.[13]

A group of teachers had started a campaign called #Teacher5aDay. It was largely facilitated through social media (hence the hashtag) but involved coordinated activities taking place in schools across the United Kingdom. It was so popular, in fact, that a national conference grew out of the initiative after less than 2 years. Their campaign centred on the five themes that emerged from a systematic review published in 2008, which looked at wellbeing across society, and how it can be improved.[14] The five themes were connect, be active, take notice, keep learning, and give. We re-deployed this as #GP5aDay (with the blessing from the #Teacher5aDay team). The key messages being that by building activities in your daily life that facilitated your social connections, kept you physically healthy, allowed you to pause and reflect on the good in your life, and enabled you to engage in acts of altruism, there was a good chance you would be better and happier for it and be more resilient to some of the factors that are believed to be contributing to the burnout of those working in general practice.[15]

Crucial to this story (although, ironically, not the campaign) is that the teachers had given out 'wellbeing bags' to their colleagues. These bags contained little messages about the campaign, and treats that were aligned to the messages, such as tea bags (to *connect* with someone over a cup or tea). Instead of leaflets further highlighting the negativity around working in health care at present, we felt the wellbeing bags offered an alternative form of campaign collateral that would help signpost key messages and resources as well as catalyse conversations when taken by trainees and shared with their peers and colleagues.

Our proposal gained support from leadership within the College. Members of staff were excited by the potential to work on something immediately tangible that could help make a difference. The campaign collateral was refined, re-designed and then piloted with trainees and early-career general practitioners, and then showcased at a meeting of college council. The feedback had been largely positive. The 'well-being bags' had morphed into boxes. The tea bags were still present, but they were now joined by a mindfulness colouring book and gratitude journal (both of which have a growing body of evidence suggesting their utility in mental health[16–18]).

Separated from the aims and messages of the campaign, an image of the mindfulness colouring book made its way into social media and trade-press. Subsequently, general practitioners across the country became enraged at the idea that they may be posted a colouring book to solve the issues that they face due to over-stretched and under-resourced workforce issues. Our objective, and morals, were questioned. The idea of the campaign was challenged. Plans to embark on a wider trial were slowed.

Amidst the negativity, however, came requests for sharing of work and ideas from other professions (law, veterinary medicine, policing) and requests from colleagues for the 'wellbeing boxes'.

REFERENCES

1. Lown M, Lewith G, Simon C, Peters D. Resilience: What is it, why do we need it, and can it help us? *Br J Gen Pract* 2015;65(639):e708–10.
2. Southwick SM, Charney DS. *Resilience: The science of mastering life's greatest challenges. Resilience: The science of mastering life's greatest challenges.* New York: Cambridge University Press; 2012.
3. Martin LJ, Hathaway G, Isbester K, Mirali S, Acland EL, Niederstrasser N, Slepian PM, et al. Reducing social stress elicits emotional contagion of pain in mouse and human strangers. *Curr Biol* 2015;25(3):326–32.
4. Peters D. The neurobiology of resilience. *InnovAiT* 2016;9(6):333–41.
5. Tyssen R, Dolatowski FC, Røvik JO, Thorkildsen RF, Ekeberg, Hem E, Gude T, Grønvold NT, Vaglum P. Personality traits and types predict medical school stress: A six-year longitudinal and nationwide study. *Med Educ* 2007;41(8):781–7.
6. Beevers CG, Miller IW. Perfectionism, cognitive bias, and hopelessness as prospective predictors of suicidal ideation. *Suicide and Life-Threat Behav* 2004;34(2):126–37.

7. Lemaire JB, Wallace JE. How physicians identify with predetermined personalities and links to perceived performance and wellness outcomes: A cross-sectional study. *BMC Health Serv Res* 2014;14:616.

8. Wallace JE, Lemaire J. On physician well being-you'll get by with a little help from your friends. *Soc Sci Med* 2007;64(12):2565–77.

9. Sales B, Macdonald A, Scallan S, Crane S. How can educators support general practice (GP) trainees to develop resilience to prevent burnout? *Educ Prim Care* 2016;27(6):487–93.

10. Brooks S, Gerada C, Chalder T. Review of literature on the mental health of doctors: Are specialist services needed? *J Ment Health* 2011;20(2):146–56.

11. http://www.dailymail.co.uk/news/article-3331748/Newly-qualified-doctor-voted-Trainee-GP-Year-hanged-worrying-failed-alcohol-test-work.html

12. Styles C. *Brilliant positive psychology: What makes us happy, optimistic, and motivated.* Harlow: Pearson Education; 2011.

13. Martyn Reah's #Teacher5aDay. https://martynreah.wordpress.com/2014/12/06/teacher5aday/

14. Aked J, Marks N, Cordon C, Thompson S. *Five ways to wellbeing: A report presented to the Foresight Project on communicating the evidence base for improving people's well-being.* New Economics Foundation; 2008. http://b.3cdn.net/nefoundation/8984c5089d5c2285ee_t4m6bhqq5.pdf

15. Doran N, Fox F, Rodham K, Taylor G, Harris M. Lost to the NHS: A mixed methods study of why GPs leave practice early in England. *Br J Gen Pract* 66(643):e128–35.

16. Emmons RA, Crumpler CA. Gratitude as a human strength: Appraising the evidence. *J Soc Clin Psychol* 2000;19(1):56–9.

17. Van der Vennet R, Serice S. Can colouring mandalas reduce anxiety? A replication study. *Art Ther* 2012;29(2):87–92.

18. Shapiro SL, Brown KW, Biegel GM. Teaching self-care to caregivers: Effects of mindfulness-based stress reduction on the mental health of therapists in training. *Train Educ Prof Psychol* 2007;1(2):105–15.

8

Interventions for burnout

DR. ADAM STATEN
The Red House Surgery, Bletchley

Despite the plethora of evidence demonstrating the prevalence and significance of burnout in doctors, there has been relatively little high-quality research into which interventions are most effective, cost effective, and acceptable to doctors to treat and prevent it.[1]

Broadly speaking, interventions can be grouped into those that focus on the individual and those that focus on the organisation. Both strategies have been shown to produce clinically meaningful reductions in physician burnout; but, in general, those that focus on organisational change have tended to show more benefit than those focused on the individual.[2] This supports the idea that burnout should be seen as a systemic problem, something that we are all vulnerable to as a result of our work, rather than something only suffered by vulnerable individuals. Accepting burnout as a systemic problem and tackling it at an organisational level also absolves the individual of any blame for the problem, whereas, arguably, individual solutions lay at least a portion of the blame at the feet of the individual.[1]

Implementing organisational change is however very difficult, suffering as it does from economic, political and pragmatic constraint; so, there are relatively fewer studies exploring the scope and impact of organisational change on burnout.[3] A few studies have ambitiously tried to combine both organisational change with individual intervention and, as might be expected, this strategy has shown the greatest therapeutic benefit.[1]

PERSONAL COPING STRATEGIES

Very few people will make it through medical school, and the early years of their training without having developed their own ways of managing stress. These will be largely dictated by personality type, experience and personal preference, but many of us have, over the years, developed coping strategies that may ultimately be inadequate to deal with the pressures of our jobs.

A study examining the personal coping strategies of doctors found that, at work, doctors' coping strategies are encompassed by five major themes. These themes included simply soldiering on through whatever work is thrown at them, talking things through with colleagues, humour, taking a time out, and simply ignoring the stress. The most popular theme was simply soldiering on, but this strategy, along with trying to ignore the stress, was associated with higher levels of emotional exhaustion. These coping strategies essentially rely on denial and therefore can only ever offer temporary relief. So, it is not surprising that they result in higher levels of burnout in the long run.[4]

Those who adopt coping strategies that rely on an element of denial fit into a pattern known as 'protective withdrawal'. Many people adopt this strategy, sitting tight and waiting for the situation to change. This is in contrast to those who seek to ameliorate the situation as 'change agents'.[4] Given that those doctors who adopt more pro-active coping strategies are least likely to burnout, these are the strategies that we should seek to encourage.

The more effective coping strategies, such as talking things through with colleagues or making plans of action, are not hard to implement into all our working lives. For example, Balint groups are commonly used during general practitioner (GP) training, with their cathartic and educational value well recognised, and yet how many of us carry this practice, even in a stripped back form, in our working lives after training?

The same study that investigated physician coping strategies at work found that the most popular coping strategies used by doctors to relieve themselves of stress at home included exercise, talking to a partner, spending time with the family, or having some quiet time alone. These were all found to be helpful and were more common than less effective coping strategies such as using alcohol to unwind or simply carrying on working at home.[5] The study therefore underlines the instinctive understanding that, to be happy and effective at work, we need a good work–life balance.

ORGANISATIONAL INTERVENTIONS

Interventions made at an organisation level include anti-bullying policies, the introduction of flexible working hours, promotion of mentoring programmes and the use of leadership programmes.[6] Introducing such programmes to an organisation of even moderate size is complex; so, the evidence base for these interventions is small, but what evidence there is suggests that they are effective.

Providing increased levels of social support, whether with mentoring schemes, peer support or simply allowing people the time to chat and engage with one another, has been shown to decrease symptoms of PTSD and depression as well as having a positive impact on physical functioning and health. Interestingly, there also seems to be a positive association between giving social support, for example, by being the mentor, and mental and physical health.[7]

Organisations such as the military and police forces now invest in preparatory training with the aim of readying their employees for the experience of stressful situations and the impact that these experiences are likely to have on them psychologically.[7] For example, British soldiers fighting in Afghanistan went through Trauma Risk Management (TRiM) training to ready them for the psychological aftermath of combat. The lessons learnt in this preparatory training were then refreshed immediately after particularly difficult incidents. This helped to normalise and validate the natural reactions to traumatic experiences, such as difficulty sleeping and intrusive thoughts, in a way that the doctrine of 'detached concern' within medicine does not.

Preparatory training is heavily based around the creation of realistic scenarios. In medicine, we already do this by role play, trauma moulages and basic life support training, but the focus is almost always on the immediate clinical scenario rather than the psychological aftermath of being involved in these stressful situations.

Some medical schools in America have set up well-being programmes for medical students. For example, in Boston Medical School, a programme centred around yoga and meditation was shown to help in promoting resilience, and curriculum changes made at the Saint Louis University School of Medicine, made with the specific aim of preventing burnout, were shown to reduce anxiety and depression amongst students. Similar programmes, with similar successes, were rolled out for new faculty members at the Medical School at Calgary University and for academic physicians at the Mayo Clinic where the programme was shown to reduce burnout and increase a sense of empowerment in staff.[8]

Just as TRiM training in the army validated post-traumatic psychological experiences, these medical school programmes normalised the expectation of stress. This helps to shift the problem of burnout from one of being an individual fault to a recognised systemic hazard.

REACTIVE INTERVENTIONS FOR THE INDIVIDUAL

As has been discussed elsewhere in this book, the experience of burnout in medicine is all but inevitable. We therefore need to have treatments to respond to the needs of those who are suffering.

There has been little study of treatments aimed specifically at burnout, but the overlap that burnout has with other mental health conditions such as depression, anxiety and post-traumatic stress disorder means that it is natural that treatments used for burnout run along the same lines as those for these other, common mental health problems.

Cognitive, behavioural and mindfulness-based interventions have all been shown to reduce physician stress and anxiety.[9] Cognitive behavioural therapy (CBT) is therefore a mainstay in treating burnout, and several studies have suggested that group, cognitive behavioural–based programmes reduce GP distress, at least in the short term.[10]

Doctor mental health programmes such as the Practitioner Health Programme in London rely on such conventional treatments to treat doctors and dentists with mental health and addiction problems, many of whom are already seriously unwell by the time they seek help.[11]

For those who need it, when there is a co-existent mental health diagnosis, then antidepressant medication and anxiolytics will also have a role to play in the management of burnout.

PROACTIVE INTERVENTIONS FOR THE INDIVIDUAL

The shift in psychology in the latter half of the 20th century towards 'positive psychology', that which seeks to enhance wellbeing rather than simply treat pathology, has spawned numerous training programmes that are designed to increase the resilience of individuals and so decrease their risk of burning out. These variations around a general theme have been researched and evaluated with varying degrees of scientific rigour.

For example, 'coaching' is something that, as yet, lacks a solid evidence base for its use amongst physicians, but it is already very popular in the worlds of business and commerce and is increasingly used in the medical profession. Coaching is aimed at harnessing the doctor's natural capabilities and helping to challenge fixed thought patterns or automatic mental responses to enable doctors to respond better to stress. Unlike CBT, it is not aimed at treating specific diagnoses: it is aimed at increasing wellbeing. It is not about getting better, it is about performing better.[12]

Training programmes that come from the same school of thought are 'hardiness training' which focuses on teaching problem-solving skills, creating supportive social relationships and changing the way people perceive stressful situations and has been shown to reduce stress and depression, and to increase performance[13]; 'stress inoculation' in which people are taught to recognise their own stress responses, are taught coping strategies such as guided self-dialogue and then practice these skills in increasingly stressful role play scenarios[7]; and 'learned optimism' which aims to change the way people perceive stress and challenge to engender optimistic thinking.[14]

As some medical schools in America are already doing, it may be that elements of these training programmes should find their way into medical school curricula in the United Kingdom and, probably, into general practice and specialty training pathways.

CAN COACHING HELP?

Richard Stevens

Former GP, Qualified Time to Think coach
Acting Director, Thames Valley Professional Support Unit

It is a great irony that the times when we most need help and support we have the greatest difficulty seeking it. This is true of many people and all the more with the medical professionals who too often equate seeking help with weakness and failure. The kindest and most generous doctors can be very harsh on themselves.

If we compare ourselves to our equivalents in other professions and in industry we can see many differences. Foremost of these is that, unlike doctors, they tend to be less embodied and identified with their jobs. In addition enlightened firms realise the benefits in protecting and developing their human 'assets' and many offer some form of coaching.

Coaching has many forms and models but, put most simply, it aims to unlock the potential within an individual and support any shifts needed to achieve agreed goals. It is often confused with mentoring or counselling and indeed it can overlap with these. Some of the skills and techniques used are fairly generic and can be seen in all three techniques – and in teaching and training, and consultation skills.

In my coaching practice there are a few beliefs that are central and axiomatic. Foremost among these is that the mind that has the problem is the mind that has the answer (and most likely the best answer for the specific circumstances of the individual concerned). There is a world of difference between being told what is the right thing to do and coming to a decision for yourself about what is the best thing for you.

A good starting place is to pose the question "what is the life you want to lead?" Implicit in this question is that we have a choice in this for ourselves – something that may seem novel to many doctors who have been through the sausage-machine that can sometimes be medical training, or who may have been unknowingly pleasing others rather making their own choices.

Only once when I have asked this question has the coachee, after thought and reflection, answered in terms other than lifestyle, contentment and work/life balance (this person, who's goal was to maximise income above all else, came from California and there may be cultural factors in play).

Although there are many different models of coaching, agreeing a shared aim or goal is fairly universal. The focus is usually on the 'here and now' and whatever skills, tools or techniques are used the flavour is of helping someone to learn rather than teaching someone.

It is commonly found that doctors prefer to engage with another doctor because they will understand what practising medicine is really like. This might be correct but a good coach will be able to empathise and understand and may be better trained in coaching than a 'member of the medical tribe'. It will be fairly certain too that non-medically qualified coaches are easier to find.

Many areas have arrangements to provide coaching to doctors through arrangements with Professional Support Units, Local Medical Committees, Clinical Commissioning Groups etc. Finding an independent coach is always a possibility too. Obviously this would require payment by the individual but this can be the best investment you ever make. It is an individual relationship so it may be helpful to shop around to get a good fit of personalities and not be discouraged if you don't gel with the first person you see.

Finally the world of coaching is still relatively under regulated and it is worth exploring training, affiliation and supervision. Personal recommendations and referrals are helpful too.

Although it seems a big step, our non-medical colleagues would not think twice about it and neither should we.

MINDFULNESS

Mindfulness is enormously in vogue, and it underpins many of the coping strategies taught in the resilience programmes described above as well as many of the therapeutic techniques used in treatments such as CBT. Type 'mindfulness' into the search bar of Amazon and it will return tens of thousands of results; yet, many doctors will only have a vague notion of what this technique actually is.

Mindfulness derives from Buddhist meditative practices, but it is considered by most of its practitioners to be non-religious and this secularity, along with a solid scientific basis, are thought by some to make it a particularly appealing form of meditation for doctors.[15]

Mindfulness has been described as a 'a form of mental training that enables one to attend to aspects of experience in a non-judgmental, non-reactive way, which in turn helps cultivate clear thinking, equanimity, compassion, and open-heartedness'.[16] It is a way of recognizing unhelpful thoughts and behaviours[15] and stopping ruminative thoughts by focusing on the present moment.[17]

Mindfulness techniques can be as simple as taking a couple of minutes to focus on a natural object around you – a tree, a flower or a cloud for example – and simply thinking about what it is that you are seeing to help clear your mind of everything else. Or you might choose to take a moment to think about a simple everyday process such as opening a door and spend that moment thinking about the tactile sensations this brings about and the physical processes involved in doing this.

There are many websites, blogs and apps from which simple mindfulness techniques can be learnt. Many of these techniques require only a minute or two to practice and so can be fitted into a busy working day. For something that is at its root so simple, there is a large evidence base supporting its use both in medical professionals and in the wider population.

Given its widespread popularity, it is not surprising that mindfulness has been studied more than any other specific intervention for preventing burnout in doctors. What is particularly relevant for the scope of this book is that mindfulness-based interventions have been studied in populations of primary care physicians.

One study explored the benefits of an abbreviated mindfulness training course on primary care physicians, with the rationale that an abbreviated course would be both time and cost efficient. Although this was only a pilot study, it suggested that the course was associated with reductions in reported levels of burnout, depression, anxiety and stress.[15] Mindfulness has also been shown to be useful in reducing stress levels in the Dutch primary care population.[18]

Mindful doctors also seem to be good for their patients. Another study found that doctors who had participated in a mindfulness-based communication program were found to have made attitudinal improvements with regard to providing patient-centred care and these changes were found to be sustained.[19]

Mindfulness is not without its critics. In particular, the claim that it is non-religious in nature is often brought into question given that many of its leading practitioners frequently make reference to the importance of *Dharma* which is a Buddhist word meaning specifically 'Buddhist teachings'. This has led some to question the ethics of the widespread promotion of religious teaching under the guise of a secular, stress reduction strategy. Nevertheless, there are clearly lessons to be learnt from the practice of mindfulness with regard to reducing our chances of burning out.

CONCLUSIONS

Despite the volume of articles and papers written on the subject of preventing or alleviating burnout in doctors, there is little high-quality research. There are still big areas in desperate need of further research such as which interventions offer best value for money, what combination of interventions may be most effective and what the long term impact of these interventions may be.[2]

What is clear however is that research into this area is gaining momentum, and clear benefit has been demonstrated from a variety of different interventions. Many of these interventions are cheap and simple to apply, and perhaps we should all be exploring which of these changes may suit us best and which could quickly be used in our day-to-day working lives.

REFERENCES

1. Panagioti M, Panagopoulou E, Bower P, Lewith G, Kontopantelis E, Chew-Graham C, Dawson S, van Marwijk H, Geraghty K, Esmail A. Controlled interventions to reduce burnout in physicians: A systematic review and meta-analysis. *JAMA Intern Med* 2017;177(2):195–205.
2. West CP, Dyrbye LN, Erwin PJ, Shanafelt TD. Interventions to prevent and reduce physician burnout: A systematic review and meta-analysis. *Lancet* 2016;388(10057):2272–81.
3. Montero-Marin J, Zubiaga F, Cereceda M, Piva Demarzo MM, Trenc P, Garcia-Campayo J. Burnout subtypes and absence of self-compassion in primary healthcare professionals: A cross-sectional study. *PLoS One* 2016;11(6):e0157499.
4. Lown M, Lewith G, Simon C, Peters D. Resilience: What is it, why do we need it, and can it help us? *Br J Gen Pract* 2015;65(639):e708–10.
5. Lemaire JB, Wallace JE. Not all coping strategies are created equal: A mixed methods study exploring physicians' self reported coping strategies. *BMC Health Serv Res* 2010;10:208.

6. Murray M, Murray L, Donnelly M. Systematic review of interventions to improve the psychological well-being of general practitioners. *BMC Fam Pract* 2016;17:36.

7. Southwick SM, Pietrzak RH, White G. Interventions to enhance resilience and resilience-related constructs in adults. In: Southwick SM, Litz BT, Charney D, Friedman MJ, editors. Resilience and mental health: Challenges across the lifespan. Cambridge: Cambridge University Press; 2011, pp. 289–306.

8. Brown GE, Bharwani A, Patel KD, Lemaire JB. An orientation to wellness for new faculty of medicine members: Meeting a need in faculty development. *Int J Med Educ* 2016;7:255–60.

9. Regehr C, Glancy D, Pitts A, LeBlanc VR. Interventions to reduce the consequences of stress in physicians: A review and meta-analysis. *J Nerv Ment Dis* 2014;202(5):353–9.

10. Murray M, Murray L, Donnelly M. Systematic review of interventions to improve the psychological well-being of general practitioners. *BMC Fam Pract* 2016;17:36.

11. Brooks SK, Gerada C, Chalder T. Review of literature on the mental health of doctors: Are specialist services needed? *J Ment Health* 2011;20(2):146–56.

12. Gazelle G, Liebshutz J, Riess H. Physician burnout: Coaching a way out. *J Gen Intern Med* 2015;30(4):508–13.

13. Maddi SR, Khoshaba DM. *Resilience at work*. New York: AMACOM; 2005.

14. Seligman MEP. *Learned optimism*. New York: Pocket Books; 1991.

15. Fortney L, Luchterhand C, Zakletskaia M, Zgierska A, Rakel D. Abbreviated mindfulness intervention for job satisfaction, quality of life, and compassion in primary care clinicians: A pilot study. *Ann Fam Med* 2013;11(5):412–20.

16. Ludwig DS, Kabat-Zinn J. Mindfulness in medicine. *JAMA* 2008;300(11):1350–2.

17. Van Gordon W, Shonin E, Griffiths MD. Are contemporary mindfulness-based interventions unethical? *Br J Gen Pract* 2016;66(643):94.

18. Verweij H, Waumans RC, Smeijers D, Lucassen PL, Donders AR, van der Horst HE, Speckens AE. Mindfulness-based stress reduction for GPs: Results of a controlled mixed methods pilot study in Dutch primary care. *Br J Gen Pract* 2016;66(643):e99–105.

19. Krasner MS, Epstein RM, Beckman H, Suchman AL, Chapman B, Mooney CJ, Quill TE. Association of an educational program in mindful communication with burnout, empathy, and attitudes among primary care physicians. *JAMA* 2009;302(12):1284–93.

9

Final thoughts

DR. ADAM STATEN
The Red House Surgery, Bletchley

DR. EUAN LAWSON
Director of Community Studies, Faculty of Health and
Medicine, Lancaster University

THE PARADOX OF MODERN MEDICAL PRACTICE

The paradox at the heart of managing burnout is the modern expectation that doctors will be cool, calm and collected. They are expected to ooze confidence in the most demanding of circumstances. Yet, a high premium is placed on the bedside manner. Patients expect their doctors to care, to be empathetic and understand their hopes, fears and anxieties. These are verging on being mutually exclusive. The neurobiological pressures do not sit well together. Clinicians need to suppress natural primitive limbic responses they experience when exposes to these situations. The changes that occur when we face these emotional pressures push us away from the empathetic approach that patients would rather experience from their clinician. The spectrum of burnout is an inevitable facet in modern medical practitioners.

BURNOUT AND STIGMA

The experiences of stress and burnout are an inherent risk to the role of being a doctor; yet, for generations we have generally tried to ignore this risk. The idea of detached concern has guided our view of how our work should impact on us emotionally. Somehow, it has always been considered possible for doctors to spend their working lives embroiled in the emotional, psychological and physical pain of their patients and walk away unbruised and undamaged by the experience.

The bulk, complexity and intensity of the workload in general practice has increased inexorably in recent years, as has the administrative burden associated with increasingly rigorous inspection, appraisal, litigation and financial accountability. All of this has heightened an already high risk of burnout, and this has been made abundantly evident by the current workforce crisis.

And yet for many general practitioners (GPs), publically at least, burnout will remain something that happens to other people. Many of us will refuse to accept that, as doctors, we are susceptible to periods of psychological vulnerability. As GPs we all spend hours of our working week helping our patients come to terms with their mental ill-health, perhaps even suggesting the diagnosis of a mental health problem to those droves of disbelieving 'tired all the time patients' who cannot understand why they are struggling with their lives. As a profession, we have bought into the de-stigmatisation of mental illness to encourage our patients to seek the help that they need, yet the stigma of mental health problems for people within our own profession is often still felt keenly.

Rather than seek help, many doctors persist in churning on, working in an ever-looping spiral of procrastination, poor decision making and callous thinking. We seek help late, often only in crisis, by which point we have compounded our problems by self-medicating with alcohol, drugs or even food.

Until we accept that stress and burnout are an almost universal experience within medicine, felt by almost all doctors at one time or another, then it is unlikely that we will succeed in creating systems and working environments in which the threat of burnout can be mitigated and within which those who suffer from burnout can readily be revitalised and returned to effective work.

THE SCIENCE OF HAPPINESS

There is a growing exploration of the factors that make people happy – their self-reported wellbeing. There is a risk that talking about the 'happy doctor' is trite and trivialising. However, the study of happiness is in many ways an easy partner with the study of burnout. It is important that mental illness and unhappiness are not conflated – a GP who is experiencing severe problems with burnout and has developed enduring mental health problems needs explicit support and therapy.

The annual World Happiness Report considers the social foundations of happiness and also outlines some of the key determinants of happiness and factors that matter in work.[1] In relation to work, people who are unemployed are in a much worse position. As are those whose work involves manual labour. Some of the factors that matter are work–life balance, autonomy, variety, job security, social capital and health and safety risks.

In many respects, working as a medical professional offers unrivalled opportunities for happiness. We come back to the underlying tension, but we also have to recognise the importance of the infrastructure in which health care professionals are working.

COMING CHANGES

The impact of burnout on the general practice workforce is undeniable and, in a National Health Service (NHS) that is built around primary care, the struggle to recruit and retain GPs threatens the very functioning and sustainability of the health care system as we know it. This realisation has finally provoked a reaction from the NHS superstructure and from the medical professional bodies that govern us.

The *General Practice Forward View* of 2016 demonstrated that there was a willingness to engage with the issue of GP burnout at a strategic level. With pledges to increase funding, reduce the administrative burden and invest in infrastructure, the *Forward View* sought to address many of the practical issues that lie at root of stress and burnout for many GPs.

Money has also been invested into services such as the 'GP Health Service' which help to tackle the problems of GP burnout, with its associated issues of depression, anxiety and addiction, at an individual patient level. The Royal College of General Practitioners (RCGP) has also produced a wide range of resources and information to help doctors who are suffering. Slowly, there is a cultural change at the top of our profession that recognises that individual burnout poses an existential threat to the whole health care system. This cultural change needs to be matched by a similar change of mindset at a grassroots level.

These changes in policy and funding bring with them the promise of change at therapeutic, cultural and organisational levels, but for these things to succeed, GPs must engage with the organisations that are now trying to provide help. GPs have real influence over the way our health service is run, whether that is by commissioning services via the Clinical Commissioning Groups, taking political action via the Local Medical Committee or engaging in the professional discourses at the British Medical Association or RCGP which will ultimately influence health policy. But unless individual GPs take it upon themselves to engage with these organisations then they will never be able to exercise the influence that they might wish for.

REFERENCE

1. Helliwell JF, Layard R, Sachs J. 7. *World Happiness Report.* United Nations Sustainable Development Solutions Network; United Nations: New York. 2017.

Index